Adel Bouguezzi

Diode Laser in Oral Surgery

Adel Bouguezzi

Diode Laser in Oral Surgery

Imprint

Any brand names and product names mentioned in this book are subject to trademark, brand or patent protection and are trademarks or registered trademarks of their respective holders. The use of brand names, product names, common names, trade names, product descriptions etc. even without a particular marking in this work is in no way to be construed to mean that such names may be regarded as unrestricted in respect of trademark and brand protection legislation and could thus be used by anyone.

Cover image: www.ingimage.com

This book is a translation from the original published under ISBN 978-620-2-53889-3.

Publisher:
Sciencia Scripts
is a trademark of
Dodo Books Indian Ocean Ltd., member of the OmniScriptum S.R.L Publishing group
str. A.Russo 15, of. 61, Chisinau-2068, Republic of Moldova Europe
Printed at: see last page
ISBN: 978-620-2-69185-7

The Diode Laser in Oral Surgery:

Dr Adel BOUGUEZZI

Preface

The history of a surgical discipline is, from its inception, marked by significant events, among which the publication of a reference book is undoubtedly one of the major elements. For diode-laser-assisted oral surgery, it must be acknowledged that very few have been published. It is a great satisfaction and a great honour to be able to preface this book on oral surgery. The chronological succession of the various chapters allows a step-by-step presentation of a logical and progressive teaching.

Clearly written and very complete in their documentation, all the most recent aspects are analysed in the light of a bibliography placed at the end of each chapter. This formatting greatly facilitates the use of the work for both the student and the practitioner. This is an essential point for the reader who will be able, if he wishes, to find or rediscover the motivations of an operating technique presented according to a rigorous chronology. An excellent and numerous colour iconography is very effective in reinforcing the understanding of the text.

Today, one can no longer practise dentistry while ignoring innovations. Each student and each practitioner must be aware of the responsibility he or she bears towards his or her patient. Forbearance from therapy therefore constitutes professional misconduct.

Reading this book will only strengthen the reader's conviction, while giving him the possibility to intervene effectively at all levels of diode laser assisted surgical therapy. A place of choice must be reserved for it in any odontological library.

Dr Adel Bouguezzi
University Hospital Assistant in Oral Medicine and Surgery
Monastir Faculty of Dentistry

Introduction

Doday, medicine has undergone an integral revolution in all disciplines through the use of new techniques and means, allowing patients to benefit from a high quality of care in optimal conditions of comfort.

The laser, an acronym for *Light Amplification by Stimulated Emission of Radiation,* has been part of this revolution since its invention in 1960.

As for their use in dentistry, and particularly in oral surgery, today laser systems are rapidly improving as they allow a wide range of treatments.

In the dental office, the diode laser, also known as a semiconductor laser, is considered a recent and particular therapeutic modality that can be integrated into most soft tissue surgeries, thanks to its exceptional incision, coagulation, hemostasis and healing performance compared to conventional surgical techniques.

The objective of our work is to present, in a first part, clinical cases on the interest of the diode laser in oral surgery.

In a 2nd part, the classification and mechanism of laser operation will be discussed and in a 3rd part, the diode laser and its different applications in oral surgery will be discussed.

❖ **Laser apparatus :**

The cases presented were carried out in the Department of Oral Medicine and Surgery at the University Hospital Clinic of Dentistry in Monastir, with a diode laser device whose parameters are :

- Elexxion pico
- Dental Laser Class 4
- Wavelength: 808nm +/- 10nm
- Maximum power: 5 W
- Pulse repetition frequency : Up to 20,000 Hz
- Pulse duration: from 26Us to CW
- Viewing beam: red (650 nm +/-5nm, max1Mw)

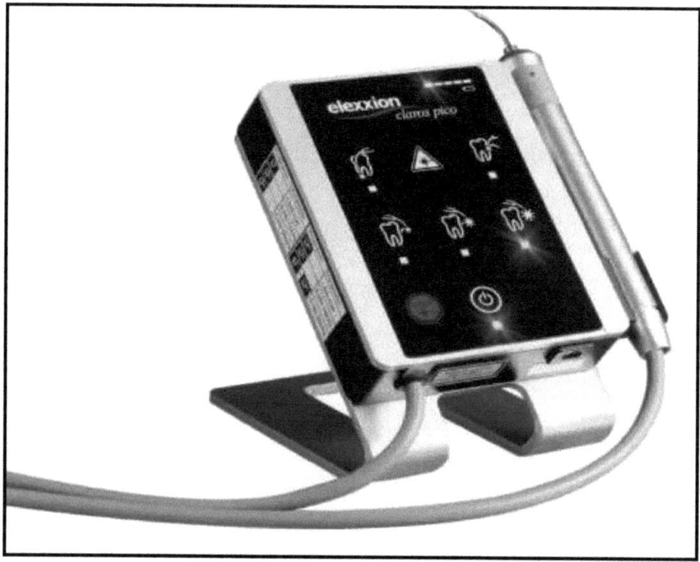

Figure 1: Diode laser "elexxion pico".

1. Gingival depigmentation

1.1 Clinical case N°1

A 22-year-old patient, of brown race, consulted the department of oral medicine and surgery at the dental clinic of Monastir with *"black gum"* as his main complaint. The patient was in good health with no medical or surgical history. Intraoral examination revealed generalized brown pigmentation of the gum associated with a decayed upper central incisor (Fig.2). Considering the patient's concerns, a laser depigmentation procedure was planned. A diode laser, with a wavelength of 810 nm, was selected for the procedure. After a local infiltration of anaesthesia, the melanin-pigmented gum was resected by laser vaporization with a flexible laser fiber emission system (300nm), with standardized protective measures. The procedure was performed on the entire pigmented anterosuperior attached gum. The remains of the resected tissue were removed using sterile gauze moistened with saline solution. This procedure was repeated until the desired depth of tissue removal was reached, combined with lip brakectomy (Fig. 3). Analgesics and 0.2% chlorhexidine mouthwash were prescribed.

No post-operative pain, bleeding, infection or poor healing occurred at the first and subsequent visits. It should be noted that a greyish-white fibrin layer completely covers the "laser" wound 6 hours after the operation (Fig.4), which was previously misinterpreted as a localized secondary infection. The result was satisfactory for the patient and the evolution was favourable (Fig.5).

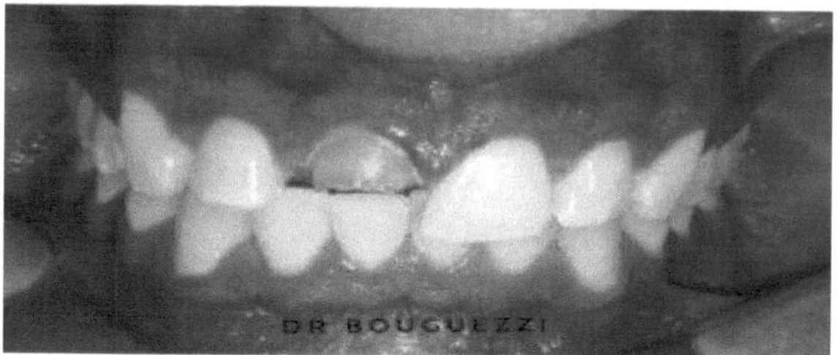

Figure 2: Pigmented aspect of the attached gum.

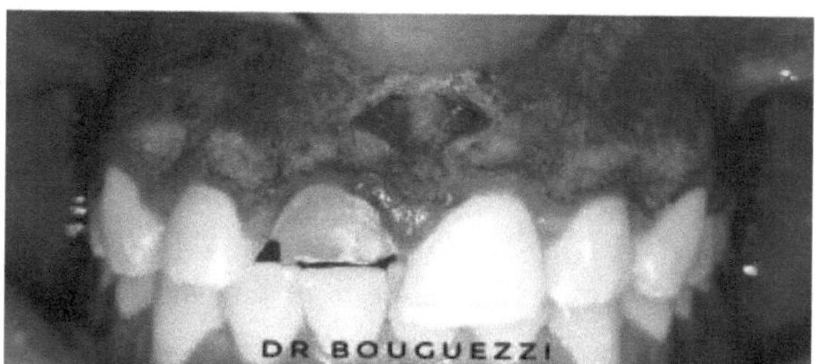

Figure 3: Immediate postoperative clinical appearance.

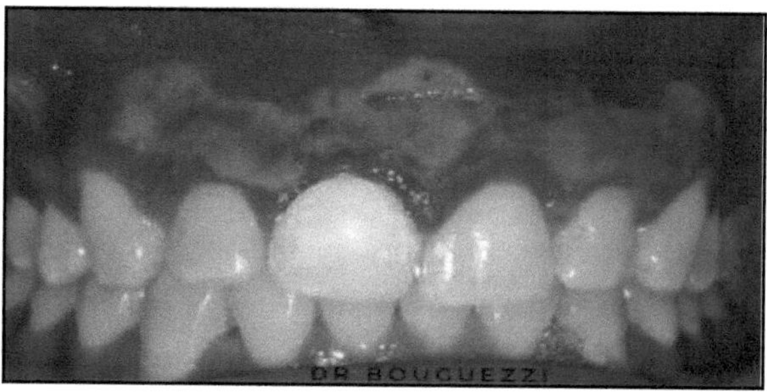

Figure 4: Fibrinous network deposition 24 hours after laser treatment.

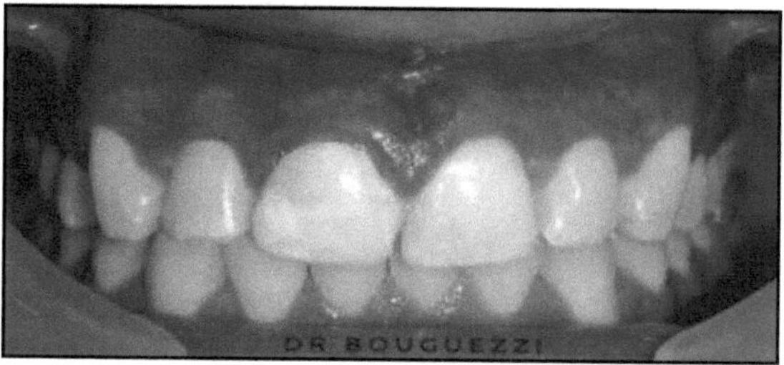

Figure 5: Three weeks postoperatively.

1.2 Clinical case N°2

A 31-year-old patient with no significant pathological history consults for purely aesthetic reasons. He wishes to be treated for gingival pigmentation, especially of the anterior gum (Fig. 6). He had a thin gum with exostoses, which led us to apply the laser in a meticulous manner while scanning the fiber in a "sea wave" so as not to expose or traumatize the underlying bone (Fig.7). Depigmentation was carried out in the same way as in the first case. Analgesics and 0.2% chlorhexidine mouthwash were prescribed. Mild discomfort and minimal discomfort were felt mainly in relation to bone exostoses and the result was satisfactory (Figs. 8 and 9).

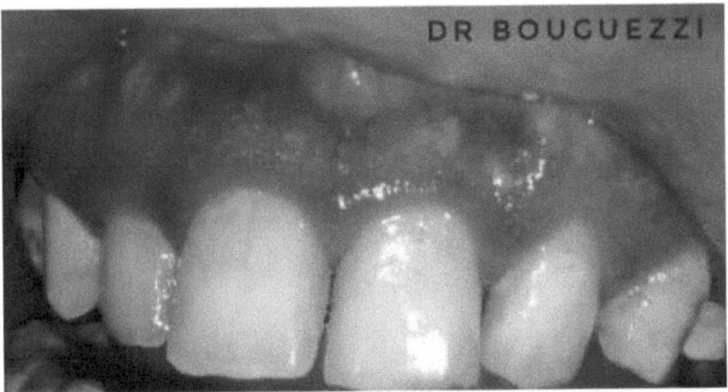

Figure 6: Fine pigmented gingiva with exostoses.

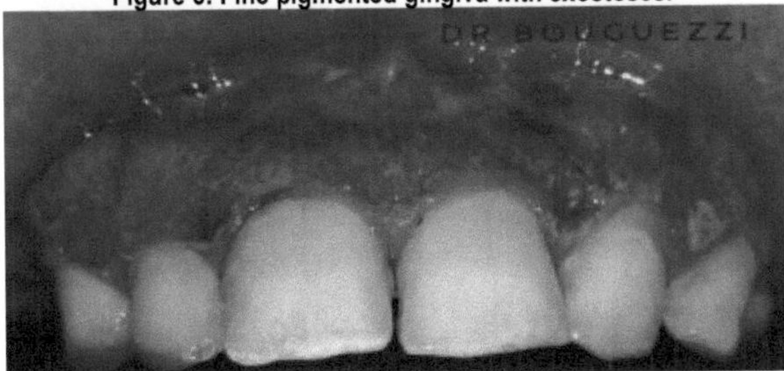

Figure 7: Laser depigmentation, immediate postoperative result.

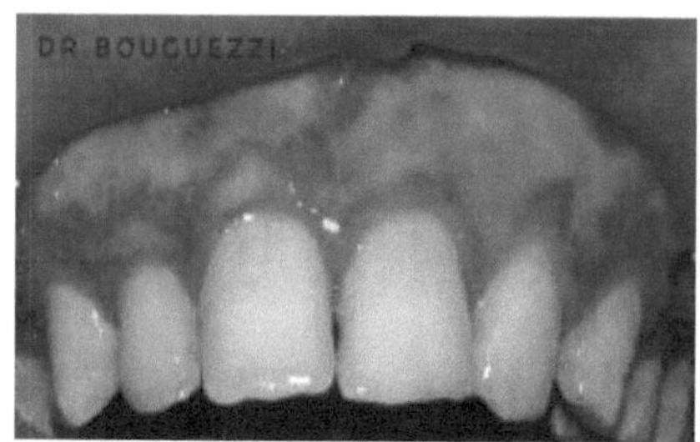

Figure 8: Fibrinous tissue network, 2 days postoperatively.

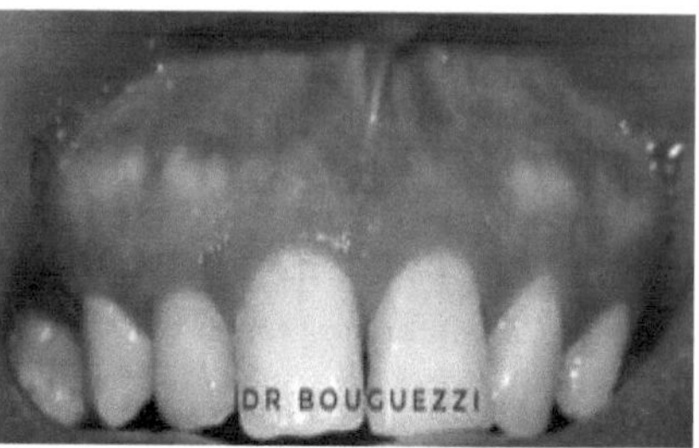

Figure 9: 1 month postoperatively.

2. Exposure of a bracket covered by hyperplastic gingiva.

A young orthodontic patient was referred to us for the management of a hyperplastic gum that completely covers the canine teeth during traction and the bonded bracket (Fig. 10). Traditional exposure with conventional scalpel surgery leads to significant bleeding and the operating field requires very little moisture, ruining orthodontic bonding on the one hand and the maintenance of good hygiene on the other. The use of a diode laser at 808 nm allowed for easy exposure with minimal bleeding and less patient discomfort. The bloodless free field allowed rapid exposure of the bracket covered by the hyperplastic gingiva for correction and management of the malocclusion (Fig.11).

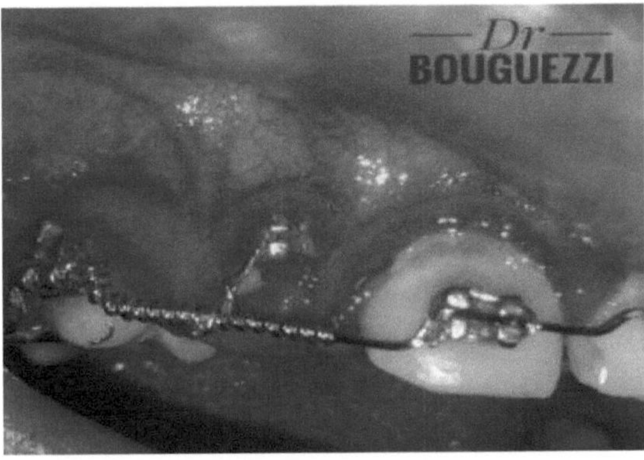

Figure 10: Hyperplastic gingiva covering the canine and bracket.

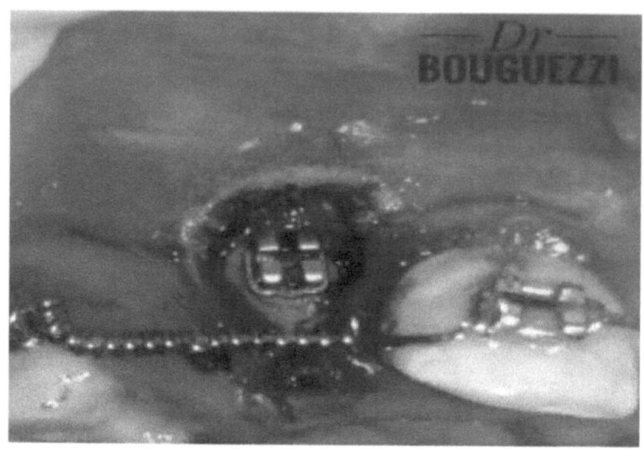

Figure 11: Bracket released by the laser energy

3. Orthodontic Dental De-inclusion

3.1 Clinical case N°1

A patient in good health followed in orthodontics for the management of a malocclusion was referred to us for the removal of an impacted canine tooth for bracket bonding and orthodontic traction (Fig.12). Canines in the palatal position are a difficult situation requiring surgical elevation of a large mucoperiosteal flap, with sutures at the end and significant postoperative discomfort and edema. The diode laser allowed exposure of the tooth without a large flap and without sutures after the procedure (Fig.13). The patient did not experience any discomfort either intraoperatively or postoperatively. The bloodless surgical field provided instantaneous bonding of the orthodontic attachment (Fig.14) and the evolution was favourable (Fig.15).

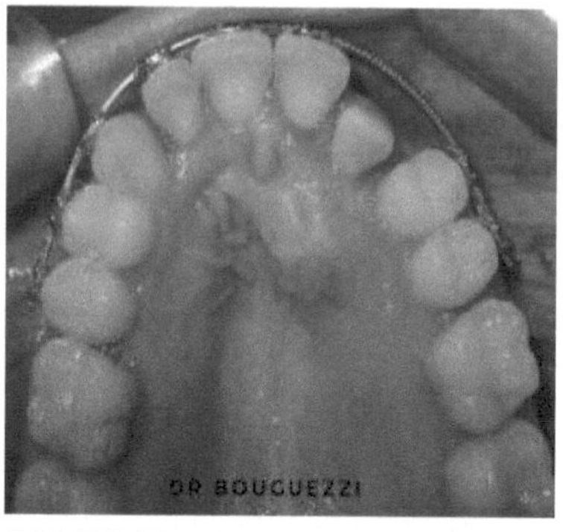

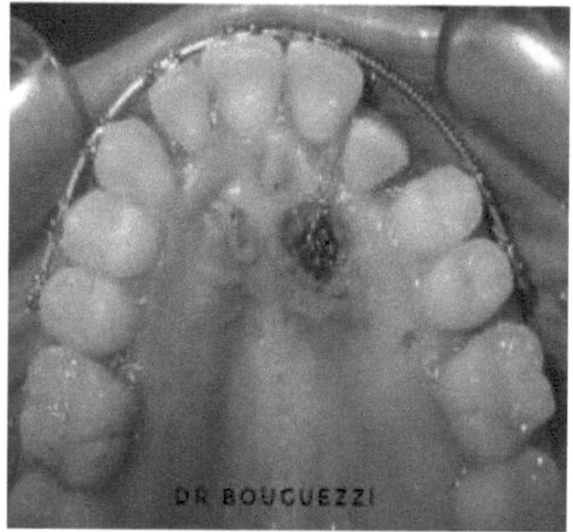

| Figure 12: Clinical aspect: Palatal voussure in relation to an included canine tooth. | Figure 13: Orthodontic attachment bonded in a dry field. |

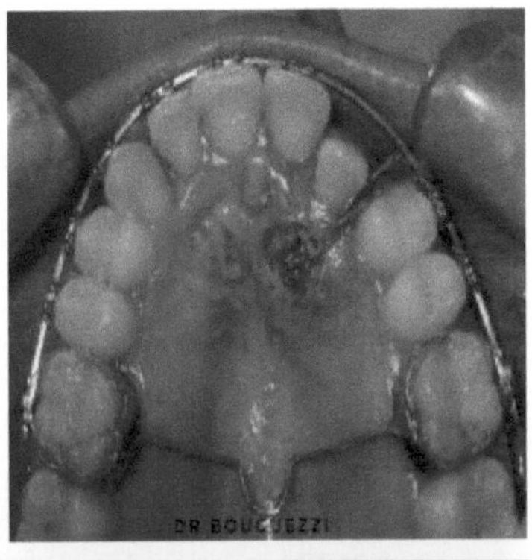

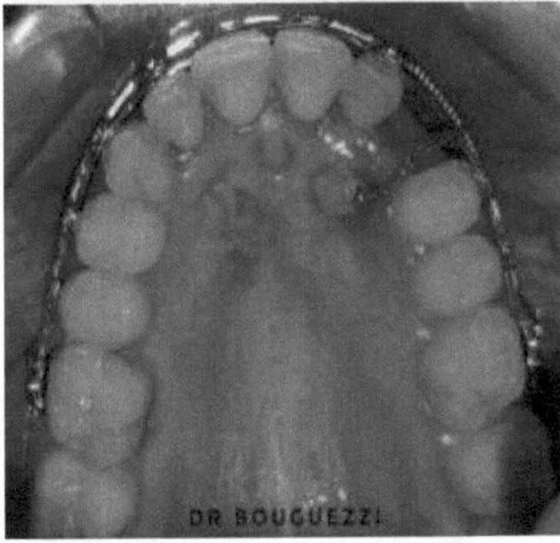

Figure 14: 24 hours postoperatively   Figure 15: Post-operative outcome at 1 month

3.2 Clinical case 2

A 17-year-old patient in good health who was undergoing orthodontic treatment for a dental malocclusion was referred to us for removal of the maxillary canine teeth under the mucosa (Fig. 16). The procedure was performed with a diode laser (808 nm, 2.5 W) and lasted 10 minutes without any intra- or post-operative discomfort (Fig. 17).

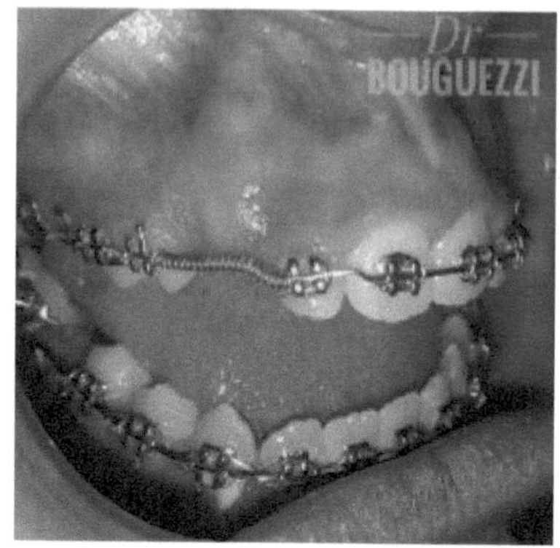

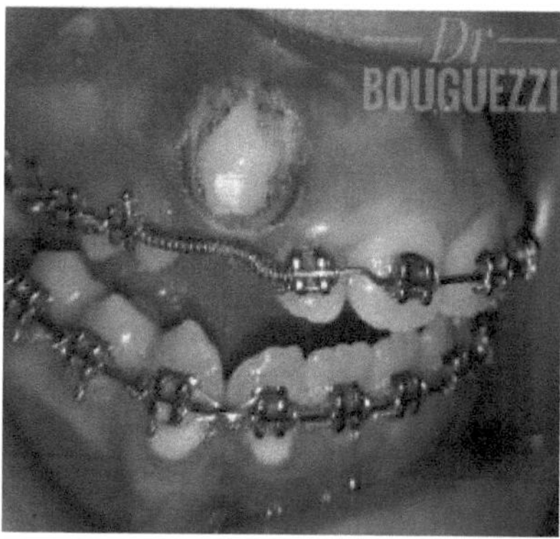

Figure 16: Canine enclosed under the mucosa.   Figure 17: Mucosal disinclusion with diode laser.

4. Labial freinectomy

After infiltrating the labial brake with local anesthetic, a traction on the lip highlights the brake which is put under tension, the tip of the laser fiber is then directed according to the incision line . The laser energy is delivered by pulse, the practitioner works in contact mode and in sea waves, that is to say by keeping the laser fiber always moving along the incision line, which is essential to avoid carbonization of the tissues and harmful effects in depth. After a complete incision, a diamond-shaped "laser" wound is obtained.

Indeed, the duration of tissue exposure is associated with the increase in temperature in situ. A cross section of the brake is made by a simple horizontal incision. It should be kept in mind that the ablation time depends on the composition of the target tissue, therefore the cross section of the brake cord may be longer than the rest of the incision. Do not shred the tissue with the fiber, let the laser energy do the cutting, in fact the laser fiber will behave like a small blade. Moreover, the power is directly related to the temperature. High powers can increase the temperature beyond the thresholds, and cause deep carbonization and coagulation in the tissues.

Sutures are usually not necessary and the wound will heal by second intention.

❖ **Clinical case**

A nine-year-old boy who had a facial trauma caused total dislocation of the maxillary inscisal area. A temporary removable partial denture is then planned for functional and esthetic purposes. Due to the low insertion of the labial brake (Fig.18), a surgical removal was performed with laser technology. A diamond-shaped extension, with deep fibre cutting, was made to avoid recurrence and tissue retraction. Excessive fibres and tissue were removed (Fig.19). Almost no bleeding occurred during the surgery, which allowed the surgeon a clear view, making the procedure quick. No coagulation was necessary. No sutures were required. The patient's compliance during treatment was very good. The treatment procedure took 8 minutes and healing was uncomplicated (Fig.20, 21).

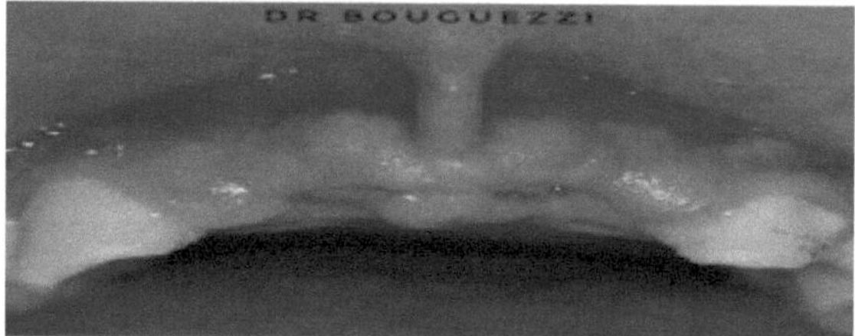

Figure 18: Preoperative situation, thick medial lip brake.

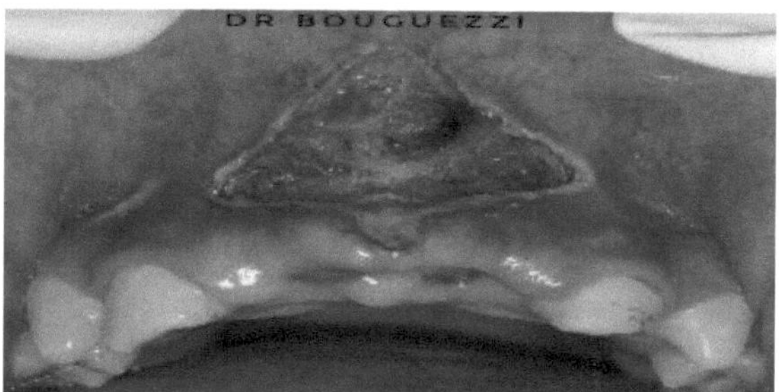

Figure 19: Immediate postoperative outcome.

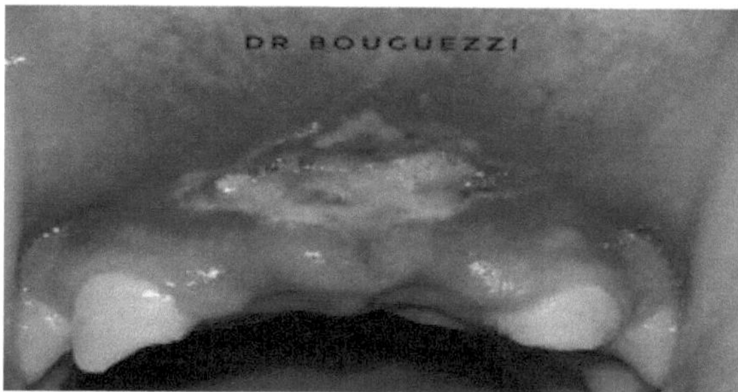

Figure 20: 48 hours postoperatively, deposition of fibrinous tissue.

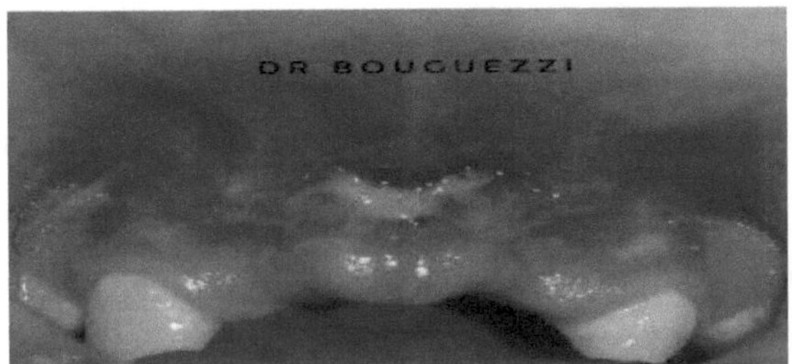

Figure 21: 15 days postoperatively.

Post-operative results after one day showed no complications. No bleeding, pain or swelling occurred. The healing process was very fast, showing a fibrin coating after one day and good vascularization; the patient was referred to the orthodontist.

5. Lingual freinectomy

Lingual laser freienctomy is more sensitive than labial freienctomy and requires very good control of the depth of penetration of the radiation into the tissue, otherwise the close anatomical structures such as the ranin bundles, the lingual artery and nerve, the salivary ducts, and the genioglossal muscles will be damaged.

❖ **Clinical case:**

A 26 year old orthodontic patient was referred to us for a lingual brakeectomy which was performed with a diode laser.

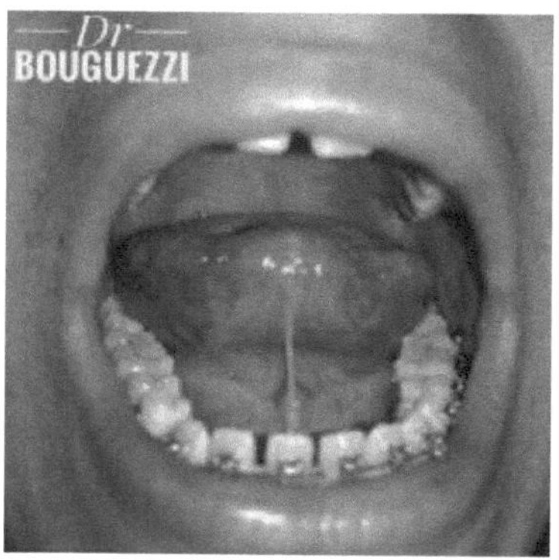

Figure 22: Initial state

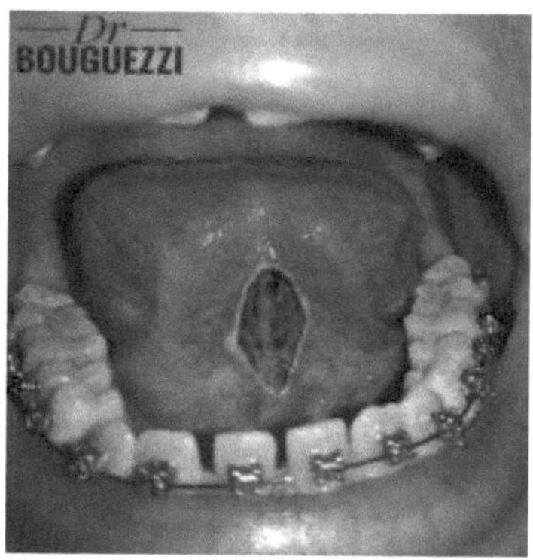

Figure 23: Laser section of the lingual brake.

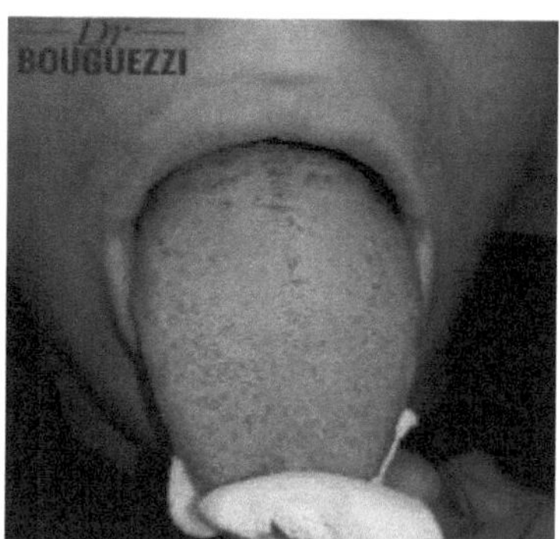

Figure 24: Result maintained at 2 months.

6. Coronary elongation associated with surgical labial repositioning

Upper lip repositioning is a simple surgical procedure designed to correct a gummy smile due to hypermobility of the upper lip. It is described as plastic surgery by Rubinstein in 1973. The goal of the procedure is to limit the retraction of the upper lip lift muscles in order to minimize gum exposure and thus reduce the gummy smile. A coronary lengthening by gingivectomy of the excess gum can also be proposed to solve this gingival smile problem.

❖ **Clinical case:**

A 21-year-old patient in good health came to the department of oral medicine and surgery at the Monastir dental clinic for purely aesthetic reasons. She wants to solve the problem of gummy smile.

The patient's medical history does not present any contraindications to surgery. Clinical examination revealed a moderate amount of maxillary gingiva on a large smile: 6-7 mm of gum exposure. The maxillary anterior teeth were short. On dynamic examination of the upper lip, lip hypermobility was noted.

At the beginning, we should check how much tissue we have to remove and how much space there is from the alveolar ridge to the top of the gum. This is done by measuring with a PA probe under anaesthesia. If the measurement is conclusive, we are able to mark the tissue to be removed. This is then useful for gum remodelling. Then we start with the soft tissue removal. In this case we used the diode laser.

Then lip repositioning surgery was performed:

Once the mucco gingival line has been located, the incision tracings have been marked and anaesthesia is administered in the vestibular mucosa and lip.

The first half thickness horizontal incision is made along the mucco gingival line. A second incision of 10 to 12 mm parallel to the first is made in the labial mucosa. Care has been taken to avoid damaging minor salivary glands in the submucosa by not spreading the lip too far apart when making the incision.

The two incisions were joined on each side by elliptical incisions allowing the epithelial band to be detached. The strip of epithelial-conjunctival mucosa was removed as a partial thickness of the

left first molar to the right first molar, exposing the underlying connective tissue.

The first stitch is medial, allowing the correct repositioning of the lip.

Separate stitches were made along the entire length of the incision in order to secure the flap as securely as possible.

❖ **Result:**

➢ Decreased gingival exposure and therefore gingival smile.

➢ Increase in the width of the upper lip, which has become more pulpy.

➢ Aesthetic results are maintained over several months.

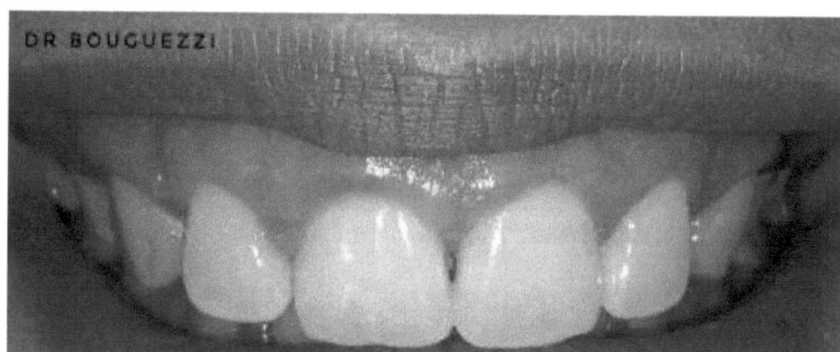

Figure 25: Gingival smile.

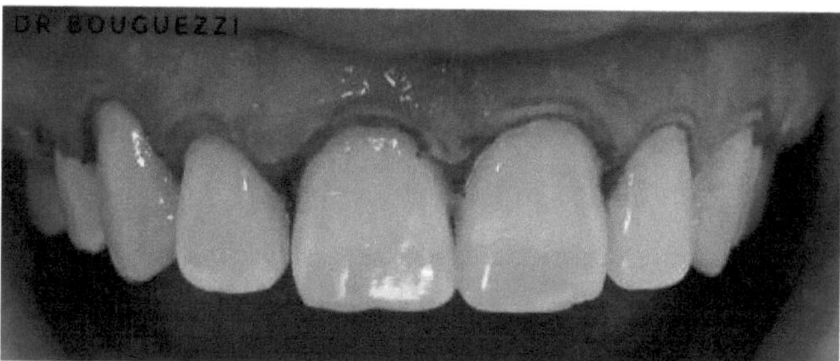

Figure 26: Coronary elongation with the diode laser.

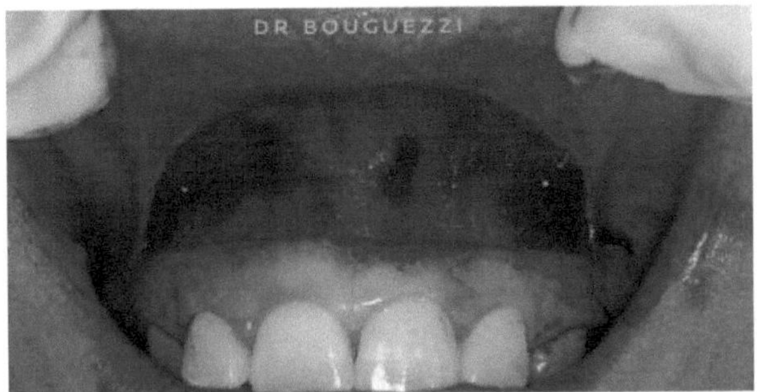

Figure 27: Partial thickness of the epithelial band detachment and exposed connective tissue.

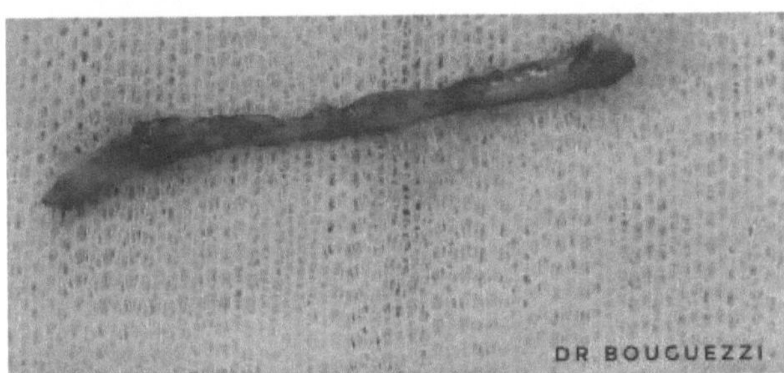

Figure 28: Epithelial band removed.

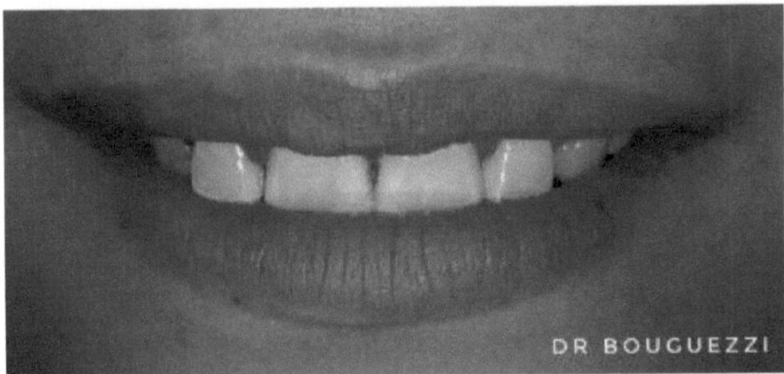

Figure 29: Immediate postoperative outcome.

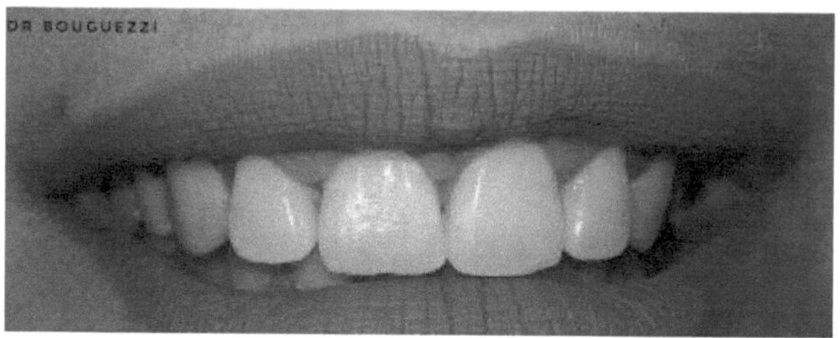

Figure 30: Healing at 1 month postoperatively.

7. Tumor exeresis

7.1. Clinical case N°1

A patient is seen for functional discomfort caused by a nodular lesion at the intermaxillary commissure (Fig. 31), with a tendency to bite. Clinical examination of the area suggests the presence of a diapneuse-type fibroid of firm consistency and 1cm in diameter. The patient's propensity to bite this region with antagonistic wisdom teeth seems to be the main aetiology of this diapneusia. The treatment plan consists of a biopsy, laser excision of the lesion and sending the sample to the pathology laboratory.

The lesion is held in place with a tweezers (Fig. 32). It is excised using the 400 μm fibre with activated tip.

The fibre, placed in contact with the lesion, is oriented tangentially to the surface of the mucosa, so as to reduce the area affected by the thermal effects of the bundle. When the radiation is activated, the practitioner must ensure that the fibre is always kept in motion to avoid tissue charring. Complete excision is quickly achieved (Fig. 33). The integrity of the lesion is preserved, and the specimen is placed in a formalin vial for histo-cytological analysis.

Biostimulation is performed by defocusing the tip of the fiber 1 cm from the target tissue so that the beam of the aiming beam covers a total area of more than 1 cm². Small circular movements are made around the lesion so as not to increase the temperature of the irradiated tissue by more than 10 to 13°. The operation lasts a few minutes, with a surgical procedure lasting less than one minute. The patient leaves with a simple prescription of mouthwash to be started 24 hours after the operation, supplemented by classical oral hygiene advice.

Anatomopathologic analysis of the intact lesion confirms the histology of a benign diapneusia.

There are no post-operative after-effects, the patient having felt no discomfort or sensitivity both in the immediate post-operative period and in the days following the operation. Healing is almost complete at the 5-day check-up. The intermaxillary region is a particularly sensitive area. Conventional surgical procedures in this area are often delicate and have disabling consequences for the patient. The possibility of intervening without side effects makes the laser a tool of choice in this type of indication.

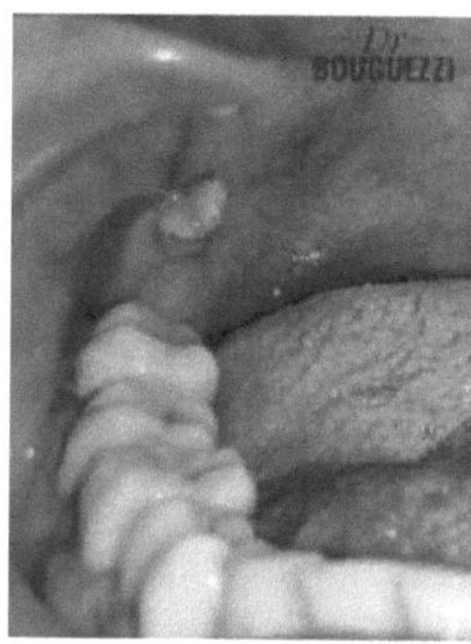

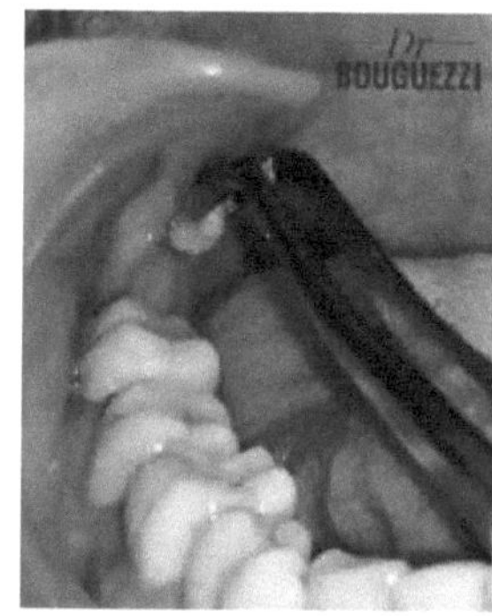

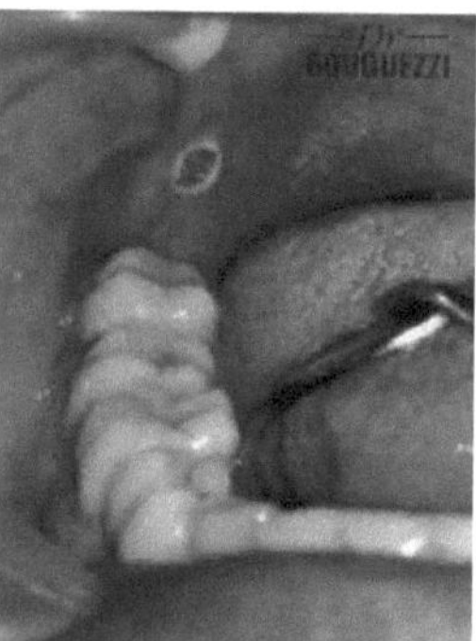

Figure 31: Nodule of the intermaxillary commissure.	Figure 32: Grasping the lesion with a tweezers.	Figure 33: Immediate postoperative appearance.

7.2. Clinical case N°2

A 44-year-old patient consulted the Department of Oral Medicine and Surgery for a nodular lesion of the labial commissure that compromised the patient's aesthetic and functional discomfort (Fig. 34). The aspiration zone opposite this nodule appears to be the etiology of this lesion. The retrocommissural area and the lower lip are rolled up as much as possible by the assistant. The tissues are then stretched at the level of the nodule and the base of the lesion more easily identifiable. The tip of the fibre is activated, the excision is performed with the activated 400 µm fibre, and the diode laser, set at 3 Watts, has allowed a precise incision to be made (Fig. 35).

Once the excision is carried out, the sample is conditioned for analysis. The sampling site, bleeding slightly, is coagulated thanks to the same fibre, creating a "biological membrane". The site is coagulated and biostimulated with the same settings as those selected for case 1. This is done to reduce the post-operative period and improve the time and quality of healing.

The pathology report shows benign diapneusia. No operative sequelae were described by the patient: absence of discomfort, pain and bleeding. The crater-like appearance obtained in the immediate post-operative period disappears within a few weeks (Fig. 36).

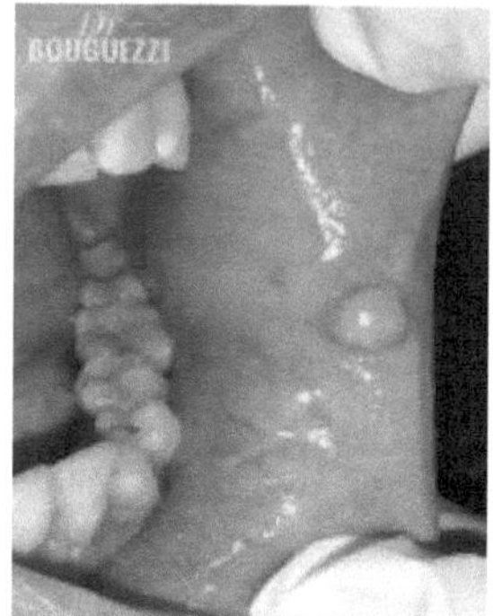 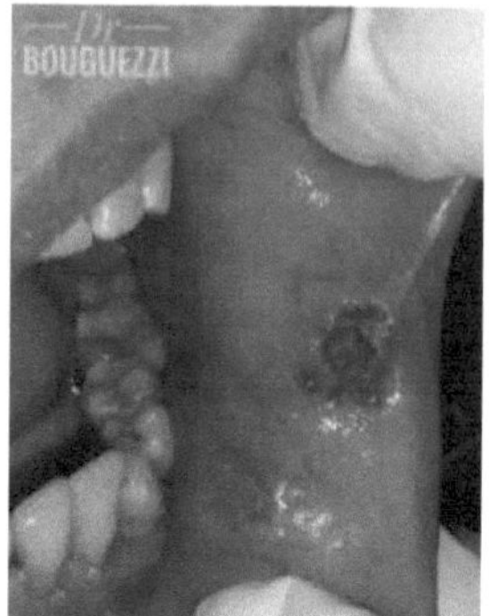

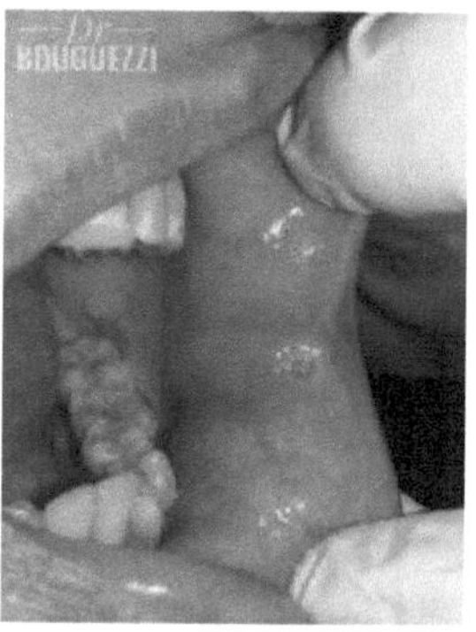

Figure 34: Nodule of the labial commissure.

Figure 35: Immediate postoperative appearance.

Figure 36: Healing at 10j.

8. Removing the cap

When the tooth is erupting, it can happen that the eruption is not complete, especially when it is a wisdom tooth. In this case a more or less important mucous cap remains around the tooth and on the occlusal surface. The laser can help to remove this undesirable mucous membrane to facilitate hygiene and to ensure better quality periodontal tissue. Here, the advantage of the laser is that the surgery is bloodless, without postoperative pain and without anaesthesia, moreover there will be no unpleasant surprises after healing since with the laser what you see is what you get.

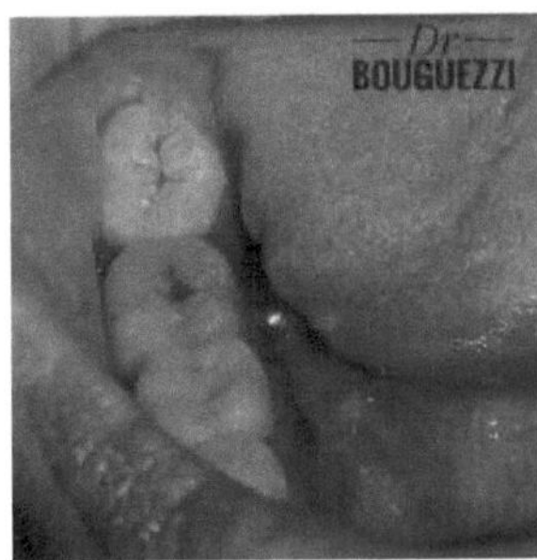

Figure 37: Mucosal cap covering the distal side of the 48.

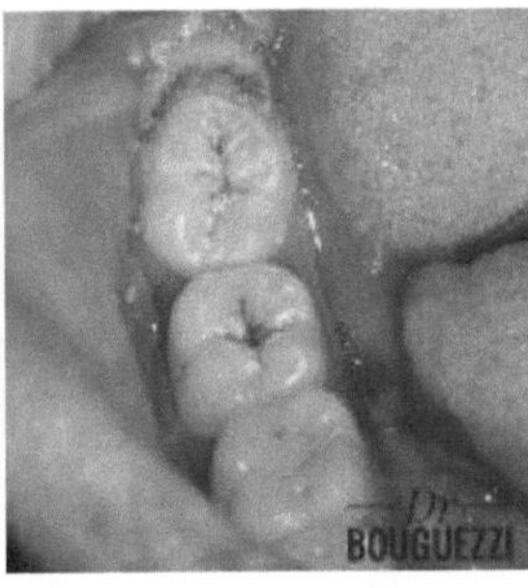

Figure 38: Non-bloody incision with the diode laser.

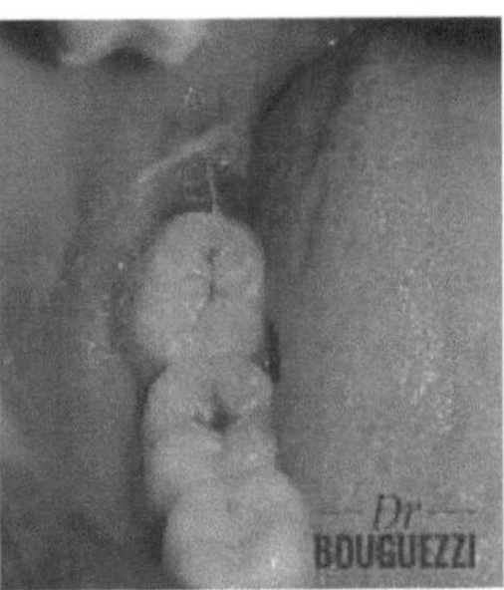

Figure 39: Healing at one week.

9. Laser and Implantology: LLLT (Low Level Laser Therapy)

A 39-year-old patient consulted the Department of Oral Medicine and Surgery for an implant to replace the 36 extracted 4 months ago (Fig.40). A suprecretal incision was made followed by drilling and decontamination of the implant site by diode laser with hydrogen peroxide (Fig.41), followed by insertion of a 4.5/11.5 implant (Fig.42). After the sutures, the soft laser (Low Level Laser Therapy) was applied using a defocusing lens with a spot size of about 1cm² to accelerate healing and minimize postoperative complications (Fig.43).

No postoperative genetics were felt by the patient.

The resulting effect of volatilization of the infiltrated tissue would also allow the biostimulation of the vascularization. The biostimulation effect increases PDGF production and bone repair. PDGF production, which normally stops on day 2, would remain active beyond the 2nd week. Revascularization would also be more intense in the treated areas.

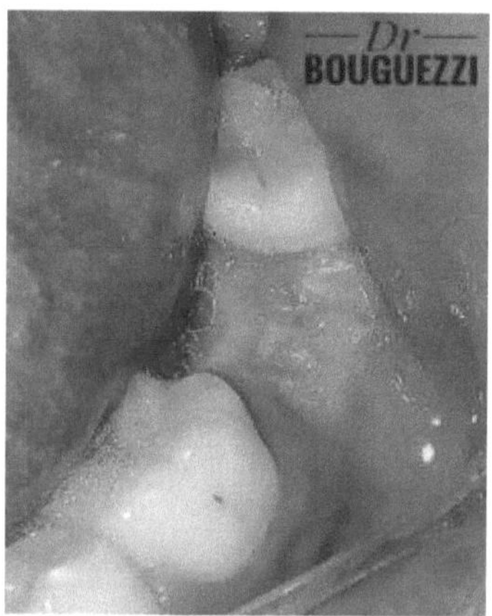

Figure 40: Preoperative clinical aspect.

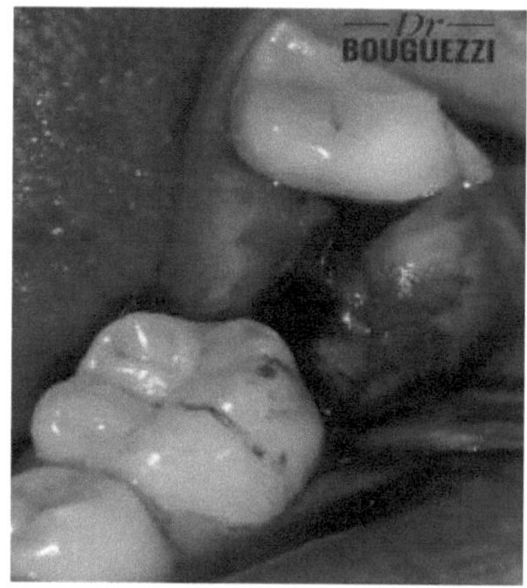

Figure 41: Laser decontamination treatment of the implant site with hydrogen peroxide.

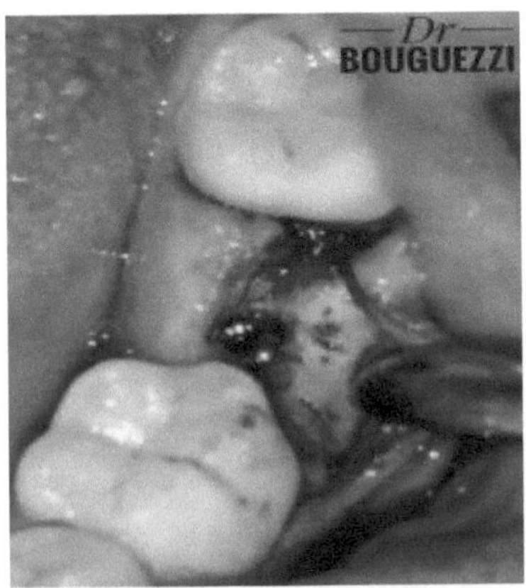

Figure 42: Implant placement 4.5 /11.5.

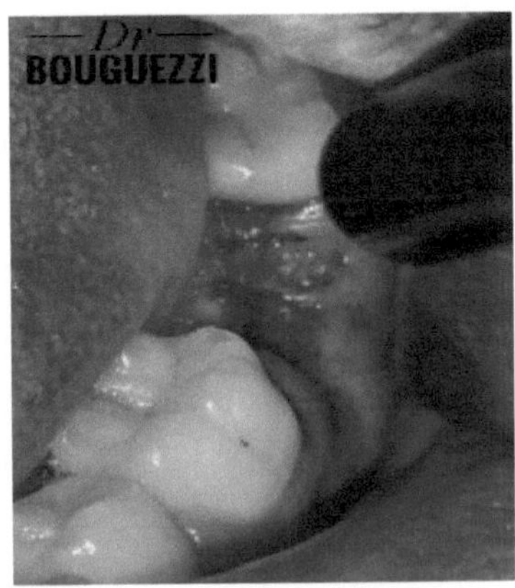

Figure 43: Low Level Laser Therapy

10. Photo-biostimulation effect

A 28-year-old patient presents in consultation with a 48 enclaved patient with a posterior marginal cystic image with the notion of recurrent infection of the pericoronary sac. Extraction was performed as atraumatically as possible (Fig. 44), followed by decontamination of the site by photodynamic therapy using a defocusing lens of the 808 nm diode laser inserted into the extraction chamber filled with hydrogen peroxide (Fig. 45).

Photo-dynamic therapy consists of the activation of a substance by radiation. In our case, the photonic energy of the radiation will be transmitted to an energy acceptor which is the fundamental oxygen that is naturally present in our cells and whose percentage is increased by the prior addition of hydrogen peroxide. The target molecules become carriers of an excess of energy, which they will transmit to the oxygen (the fundamental oxygen present in the target tissues). This photonic energy is at the origin of the transformation of the fundamental oxygen into singlet oxygen. The singlet oxygen (diamagnetic oxygen) has a lifetime of the order of microseconds and isomerizes into triplet oxygen (paramagnetic oxygen), which has a lifetime of the order of milliseconds. The triplet oxygen then falls back to the fundamental oxygen molecule available for further photonic excitation.

Then an X-shaped suture was made to bring the edges closer together and close the alveolar site (Fig. 46), followed by a second application of the photodynamic laser (Fig. 47) to potentiate mucosal healing and minimize postoperative sequelae.

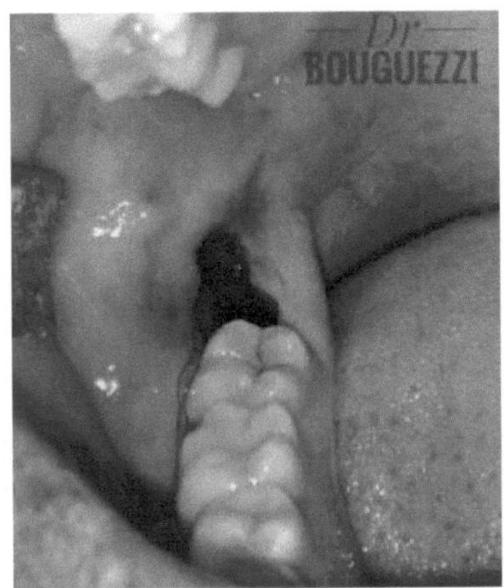

Figure 44: Post-extraction alveolar site

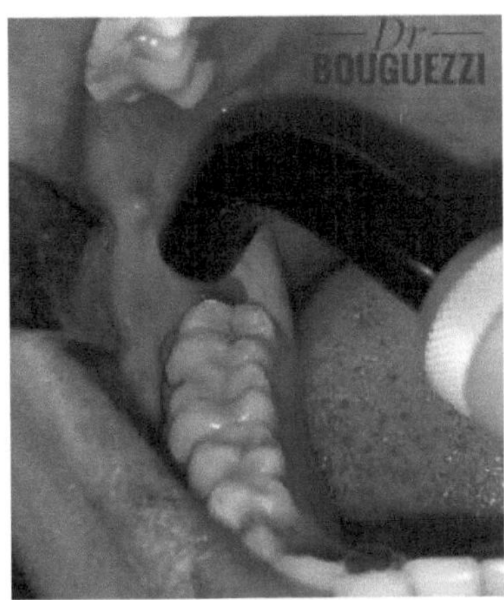

Figure 45: Decontamination and biomodulation
with the low-power laser.

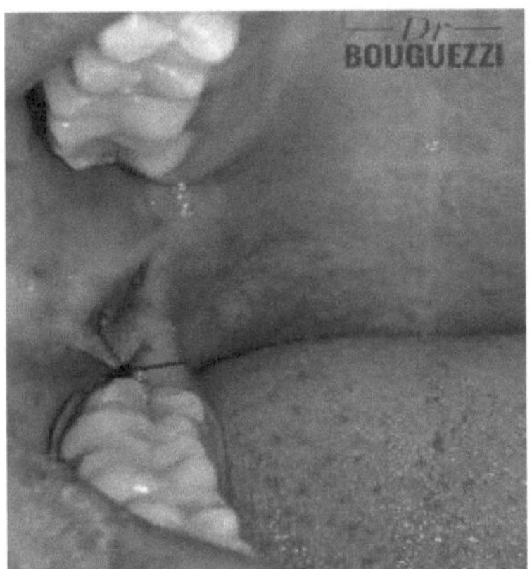

Figure 46: X-ray sutures.

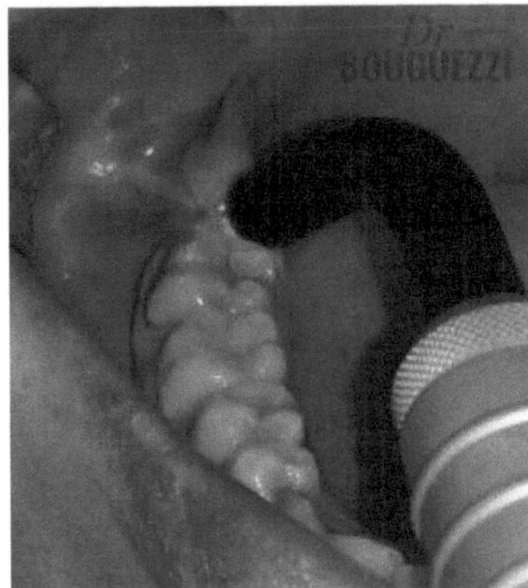

Figure 47: Second application of the low-power
laser.

11. Vestibuloplasty

A 37-year-old patient consulted us for the management of a facial asymmetry due to significant postoperative jugular tension following the closure of an oral sinus communication that occurred during the extraction of an impacted maxillary wisdom tooth with a jugular flap by a maxillofacial surgeon.

On exobuccal examination, there is an apparent facial asymmetry associated with a "hollow" cheek with significant aesthetic damage. In the endobuccal, a fibrous jugal tendon is inserted at the top of the maxillary crest which prevents the maintenance of good oral hygiene and aggravates periodontal recession of the adjacent molar.

The procedure was to clear the ridge by subtraction with a diode laser. Anaesthesia was abundant in order to fill the periodontal tissues with fluids and limit the diffusion of heat and bleeding. A finger is applied to the free gingiva at the muco-gingival reflection line with support on the bone: mesial to distal movements indicate the location of the incision. Care must be taken to firmly tension the fibromucosa during the incision, to regularly remove the calcined tissue with a curette and to irrigate abundantly. Laser vestibuloplasty is a less cumbersome procedure than grafting. The execution is faster, the result is almost immediate and the after-effects are negligible.

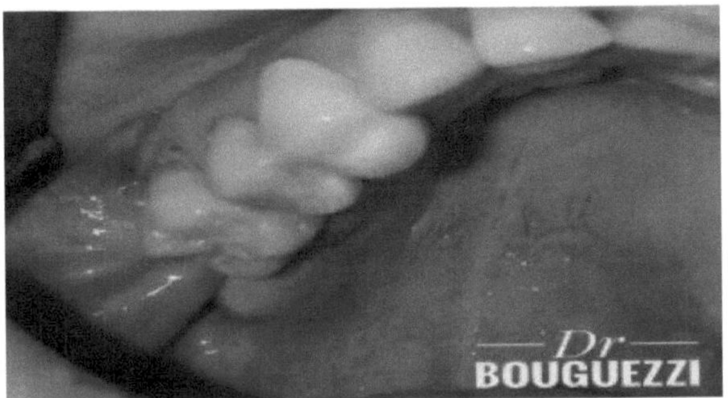

Figure 48: Jugal fibrous tendon connecting the cheek to the alveolar crest, associated periodontal recession of the first molar.

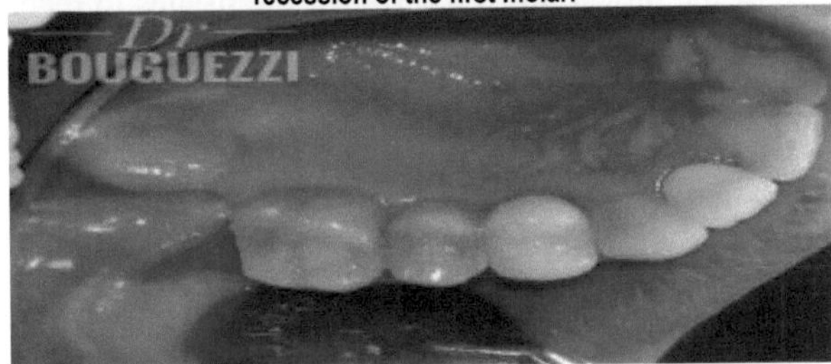

Figure 49: Supracrestal fibrous tendon that suppresses the vestibule.

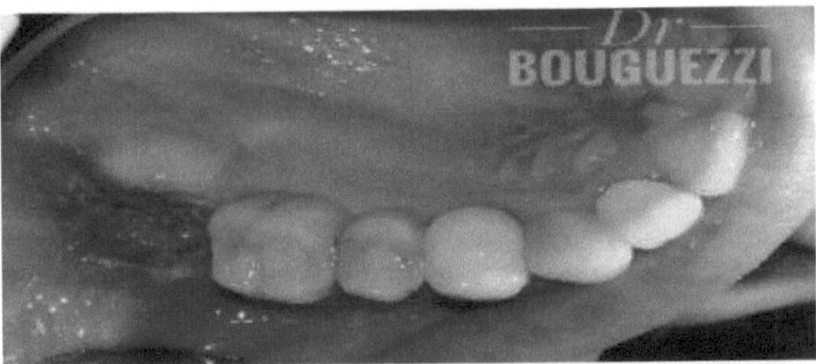

Figure 50: Tendon excised with the laser associated with vestibular deepening.

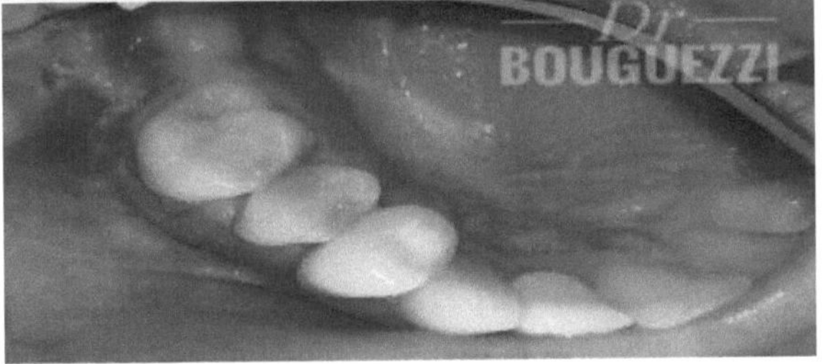

Figure 51: Healing at 3 weeks. Ridge is clear.

12. Vestibular deepening

Two totally edentulous patients who were candidates for total prosthetic rehabilitation were referred to the Department of Oral Medicine and Surgery for vestibular deepening and management of a floating mucosa.

On clinical examination, we note a very low muco-gingival line. This situation limits prosthetic stability, all the more so as the ridges are floating, especially for the 2nd patient.

The objective of the procedure is to arrange the tissues to receive an assistant prosthesis that will be more stable on larger mucous membranes.

We surgically repositioned this entire fibro-muscular assembly apically. As a result, the prosthetic contact surface will be increased and the prosthetic limits will be at a distance from the destabilizing muscle forces.

Anaesthesia will be abundant to fill the periodontal tissues with fluids and limit the diffusion of heat and bleeding. For the 2nd patient, we first treated the floating ridges by tissue sculpture on the mobile mucous membranes. This microsurgical approach allows us to regularize the ridge in a minimally invasive way associated with a brakeectomy by micro-ablation of the fibrous insertions. We then accessed the muscle structures by fine dissection and apical repositioning.

The cold blade is considered the most accurate instrument for making surface incisions on epithelial layers. However, this classical surgical technique of vestibular deepening has been widely described, but has been largely abandoned due to the relative complexity and the more than random nature of its results (recurrences). The Laser, on the other hand, will express all its potential for precision, efficiency and operative ergonomics for deep plane dissection.

By micro-ablation using laser energy, we can selectively dissect the different tissue planes with a precision of a few tens of microns per second. Here we can see perfectly the muscle layer that is to be disinserted on one side of the surface epithelial mucosa and on the other side in depth of the periosteum. In order not to lose part of the gain obtained, the vestibular repair is always associated with the insertion of a transition prosthesis to ensure modelling.

This procedure is bleed-free, allowing perfect visual control of the incision areas, thus making the results more predictive, while simplifying the clinical procedure, which takes only 10 to 15 minutes. The use of a healing guide facilitates and improves the healing process and makes the result long-lasting.

❖ **Clinical case:**

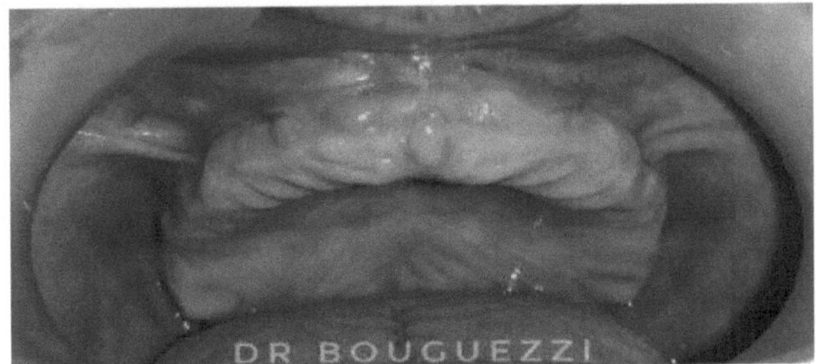

Figure 52: Preoperative condition: 2 side brakes.

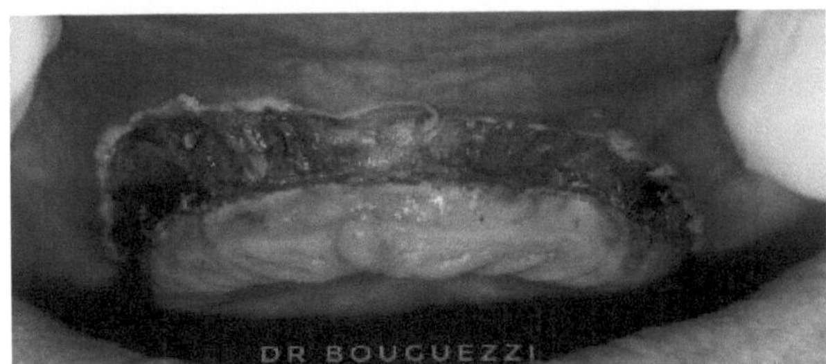

Figure 53: Immediate postoperative outcome.

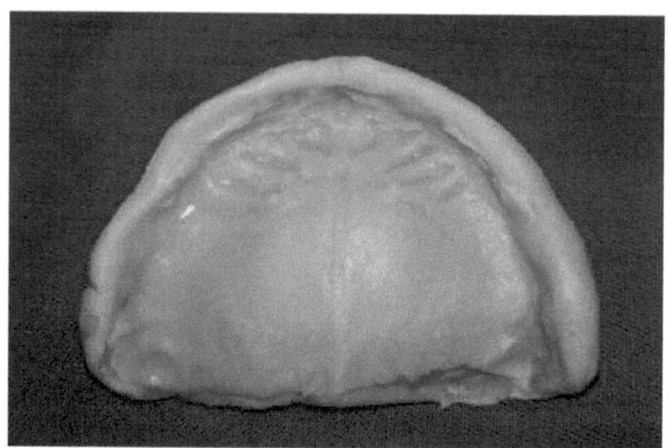

Figure 54: Total prosthesis to be used as a healing guide.

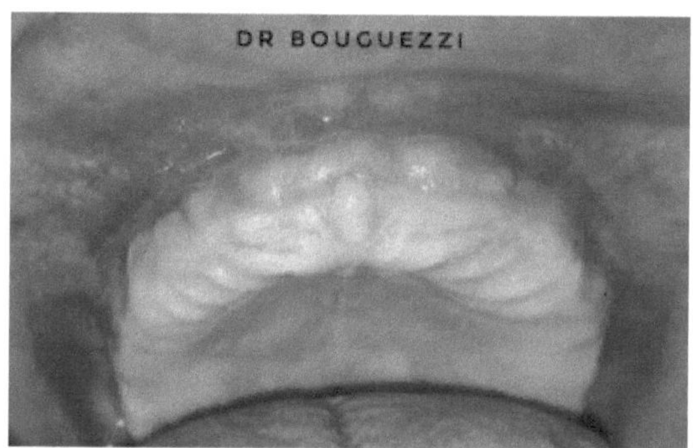

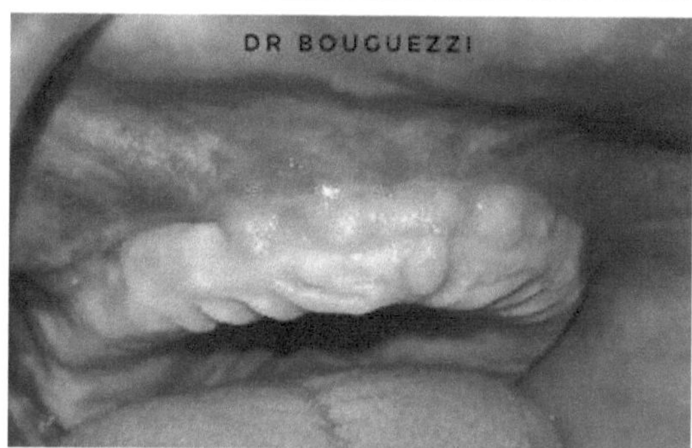

Figure 55 Figure 56: Mucosal healing after 2 months.

1. What is a laser?

It is an acronym for "Light amplification by stimulated emission of radiation". So, it is a transformation of an energy (electrical...) into a light energy with specific properties emitting in the ultra violet, visible or infra red optical radiation range, a monochromatic radiation beam (having a defined wavelength) and coherent (the waves that make up the beams are in phase). [49,52]

2. Laser classification

2.1. Classification of lasers based on power

2.1.1. High-power lasers, hot or hard lasers [4].

These are lasers for surgical use, taking the name of surgical lasers.

These lasers act on the tissues by its thermal effect. They cause necrosis, carbonization, coagulation and denaturation of proteins. It is possible to benefit from one or more of these effects by controlling the temperature produced.

The power of these lasers is usually more than 500MW. These types of lasers find these applications in surgery.

The most widely used are the CO2 carbon dioxide laser, the Nd:YAG laser and the Argon laser.

2.1.1.1. CO2 carbon dioxide laser [36,43,45,49].

The active medium of this gas laser is carbon dioxide CO2. The wavelength of 10600 nm places it in the infrared plus liontain and allows it an excellent absorption in soft tissues.

It is one of the lasers of choice for soft tissue surgery for aesthetic or functional purposes (gingival papilla shaping, wisdom teeth decapping, coronary elongation by gingivectomy, etc.).

It allows to perform effective bloodless surgery with little pain, without sutures (so no bridle) and with very good healing.

It is strongly absorbed by water and hydroxyapatite.

The major disadvantages of the CO2 laser are its large size (it is not ergonomic), its high cost and especially its destructive thermal effect on hard tissue.

2.1.1.2. Erbium family lasers (Er:YAG and Er,Cr:YSGG) [36,49]

For this type of laser, the wavelength of its radiation is at a maximum peak absorption of water and hydroxyapatite (2940nm). This laser therefore has a very low transmission with a very high immediate tissue absorption.

It will therefore be very effective on hard tissue and will even allow the removal of decayed dentinal tissue or bone surgery (sampling, crest extension...).

But they don't provide hemostasis as effectively as the CO2 laser.

Some indications for Erbium lasers: brakeectomy, removal of benign tumours (epulis, fibroma, papilloma...), apical resection, osteoplasty, bone sampling, drilling in implantology...

2.1.1.3. Nd-YAG laser [36,43,45,49]

Widely used in medicine, the Nd-YAG (Neodymium Yttrium Aluminum Garnet) laser is composed of a bar of neodymium-doped yttrium aluminum garnet crystal. It emits with a wavelength of 1064nm, therefore in the infrared. Its radiation, poorly absorbed by water, is one of the most penetrating in soft tissues (up to 10 mm and beyond), which will allow it to have a deep decontaminating action.

Its wavelength strongly absorbed by the pigmented tissues makes it a very effective surgical tool for the ablation of haemorrhagic tissues with good haemostasis. In addition, there has been research into its use for non-surgical sulcus debridement in periodontal disease.

2.1.1.4. Argon laser [39,43,45].

- The active medium is Argon, which is a gas.
- The argon laser produces light in the visible spectrum (blue-green to yellow-orange) that is easily absorbed by pigmented tissues (rich in hemoglobin, melanin and other dark pigments).

- Thus, these lasers are useful in the treatment of pigmented lesions and vascular abnormalities.

- Argon laser therapy is currently the treatment of choice for dermatological lesions.

2.1.2. Lasers with moderate powers [4]

These lasers express their therapeutic effects without inducing much heat. Their light has a stimulating effect on tissue. The power of these lasers is between 250 and 500 MW.

2.1.3. Low-power lasers, or cold lasers [4].

Also say soft lasers. They are intended for mild therapeutic applications. It is a form of therapy that uses the red and infrared light of the laser.

These lasers have no thermal effect on the tissue unlike (hot) surgical lasers, whose mode of action is essentially thermal. Its light and progressive reactions on the tissues are called **"photo-biostimulation"**.

The power of these lasers is usually less than 250 MW.

The best known cold lasers are the diode laser and the Helium Neon laser.

2.1.3.1. Helium Neon Laser [36]

It's one of the first lasers available. This gas laser is a mixture of Helium and Neon emitting a wavelength of 633nm, i.e. in visible red light.

Soft helium neon lasers provide a trophic effect by cell biostimulation, an anti-inflammatory effect and an analgesic effect.

2.1.3.2. Diode laser [32,41,49].

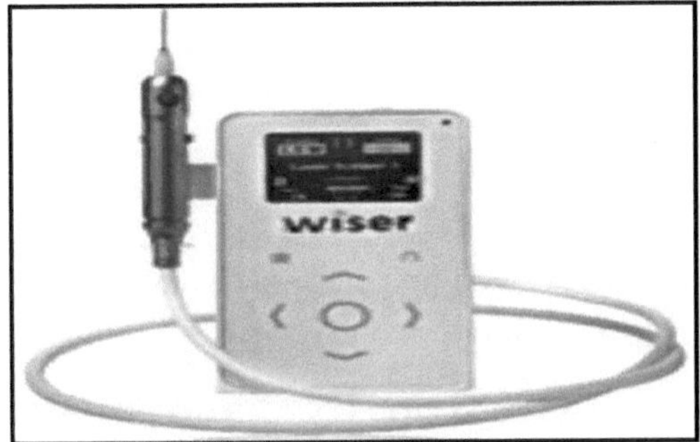

Figure 57: Wiser diode laser 980 nm. [32]

It is a recent development in the medical field. They are semiconductor lasers, of visible wavelength, widely used.

The energy is distributed through optical fibres, usually 200 or 300 um long.

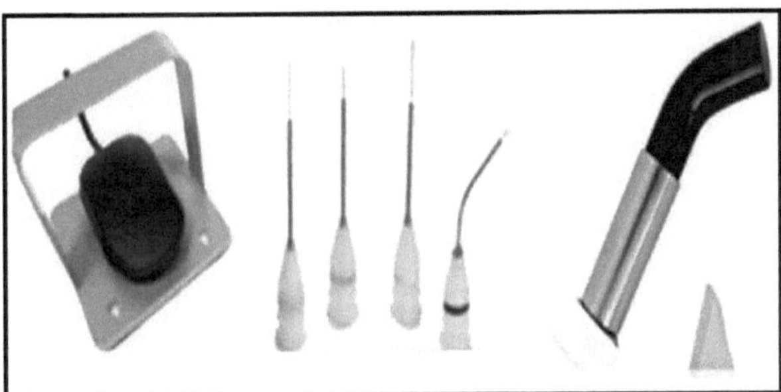

Figure 58: Foot pedal, fibers available as a tip and defocusing bent lens of the diode laser. [32]

Its light beam has a high tissue penetration (4 to 6 mm) with good absorption by the pigmented tissues.

Some diode laser indications: small vessel hemostasis, soft tissue surgery, peri-implantitis treatments...

2.2. Classification of lasers according to the active medium [4].

- **Gas lasers:** these are lasers with an electric pumping system such as CO2 laser, helium neon laser.
- **Liquid lasers:** such as dye lasers
- **Solid-state lasers:** also known as insulation lasers such as Nd:YAG lasers and diode lasers.

2.3 Classification of lasers according to wavelength [4].

Lasers are classified into 4 categories according to their wavelengths:
- Ultraviolet: 300 to 400 nm.
- Visible light ranging from 400 to 700 nm.
- Near-infrared laser: 700 to 1200nm.
- Laser far from infrared: more than 1200nm.

3. Physiological effects of lasers at the tissue level [4,20].

Following laser treatment, the tissue response can be divided into two categories:

3.1. A primary response

Vasodilatation, increased blood flow and lymphatic drainage, decreased neutrophil and fibroblast activity, accelerated cell metabolism and decreased pain threshold.

3.2. A secondary response

The decrease in the concentration of certain prostaglandins such as PGL2 which has anti-inflammatory effects, a decrease in immunoglobulins and lymphokinins and these actions in the immune system, a decrease in endorphin B and encephalins which have an analgesic effect.

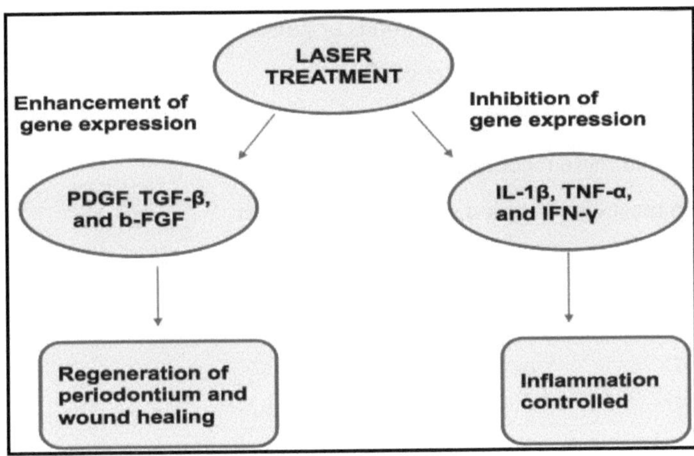

Figure 59: Physiological effect of laser therapy: regeneration and healing of pleasures with control of inflammation. [20]

1. Representation [5,20,41]

The feasibility of laser emission within a semiconductor was demonstrated experimentally in 1962 in gallium arsenide (GaAs), giving rise to diode lasers. Indeed, Galium (Ga), Arsenide (Ar), Aliminium (Al) and Indium (In) are elements that convert electrical energy into light energy. Therefore, they are used to build these diode lasers.

This type of lasers can be defined as aluminium-doped gallium arsenide diodes, thus taking the name **"Indium-Gallium-Arsenide (InGaAs)"**.

These lasers are also called semiconductor lasers, where the stimulated substance is a semiconductor called a laser diode array.

Basically, the diode laser has a construction similar to semiconductor diodes. The enhancement of the light radiation results from the passage through two adjacent semiconductor layers, called the conduction band and the valence band; one of the bands has an electron excess (n-type doping) and the other an electron deficit (p-type doping). The distance between the energy bands and their widths are determined by the selected crystal.

The diode laser is used in continuous or pulsed mode.

It is one of the visible wavelength lasers.

It is a universal laser that acts on soft tissue at three wavelengths: 980nm, 810nm, and more recently 940nm.

But the most common is the 810 nm diode laser.

1.1. The specificity of the diode laser

[20,41,46].

These are lasers that have only recently appeared in medical fields.

Thanks to the efficient coagulation, the good visual control of the laser-tissue interaction, the relatively low level of pain, the reduction to a minimum of the instruments required for the operation and the limited trauma to the surrounding tissue, the diode laser lends itself to simple and universal use.

The diode laser is well absorbed by the haemoglobin-rich tissue and allows for a better incision and good tissue coagulation.

They are strongly absorbed by pigmented soft tissues (rich in melanin and haemoglobin) giving them excellent haemostatic characteristics. However, they are poorly absorbed by hard tissue such as dental tissue, which allows surgery to be performed close to enamel, dentin and cementum without the risk of iatrogenic damage.

It can induce tissue photostimulation during surgery.

This energetic stimulation seems to improve the healing process and reduce postoperative after-effects. The patient feels greater comfort and healing is faster and more stable.

1.2. Diode laser in the dental office [41,50]

Laser technology has always been expensive. The manufacturing costs are high and the materials used to cut fabrics are very expensive. Diode lasers, on the other hand, are less expensive to produce and become available to the general dentist.

It is ergonomic and unobtrusive in the dental office (it can be easily moved from one chair to another). It is autonomous, not needing to be connected to a water or air source. The operating tip opens with a simple optical fibre. The device has several presets. The power and frequency are easily adjusted according to the operating site and the type of procedure.

The soft-tissue diode laser has quickly become a "plus" in the general practitioner's standard equipment. The technology, ease of use and price make it easy to integrate into a dental practice. It is becoming the "handpiece" for soft tissue.

Thanks to these fine fibres, it allows us to perform not only special geometry cuts with punctiform ablation, but also special minimally invasive interventions in the field of intraoral surgery.

1.3 Comparison with CO2 laser systems [41].

The diode laser is characterized primarily by its high degree of efficiency, which results from the direct conversion of electrical energy into optical energy, and by its modest external dimensions. Expensive external cooling devices, which are indispensable for other types of lasers such as the CO2 laser, are not required.

At the tissue level, it is above all the narrowness of the thermal lesion band that is remarkable, even in deep cuts.

The vertical extension of the tissue trauma, as well as its horizontal extension, is not dependent on the diameter of the optical fibre used nor on the mode of use (continuous or pulsed).

This property of the diode laser distinguishes it from the clinical results obtained with the CO2 laser and the Nd:YAG laser as well. Indeed, for these two types of laser, thermal damage to the surrounding soft tissue is much more pronounced than in pulsed mode.

During soft tissue excision by CO2 laser, superficial carbonization of the deep alveolar bone has already been reported. For this reason, in any CO2 laser procedure involving the remodeling of thin gum tissue, care must be taken to spare the bone and minimize the duration of exposure to the laser beam to avoid bone necrosis with subsequent sequestration. Of course, the pulsed diode laser with the corresponding power can in principle also cause similar thermal damage to hard tissue. However, the accidental risk of such damage during soft tissue surgery is considerably lower.

2. Application of diode laser to soft tissue in oral medicine and surgery

Thanks to the progress made in the use of the laser at the oral level, the diode laser seems to be a promising method, thanks to it, surgery becomes simpler, more reproducible and much more comfortable for the practitioner than for the patient compared to other conventional techniques.

2.1. Flange and brake surgery

2.1.1. Definitions [13]

2.1.1.1. The brakes

These are anatomical structures devoid of muscle fibres, consisting essentially of a very dense network of connective fibres as well as oxytalan fibres and loose connective tissue. These brakes, by their insertion, can generate the appearance of a certain number of problems such as the appearance of diastemas especially between the two upper central ones if the labial brakes are very low located which is disgusting for young patients, as it can be at the origin of the appearance of recurrences after heavy orthodontic treatment. As for the lingual brake, it can be the cause of ankyloglossia which limits the free movement of the tongue and as a result of speaking difficulties.

2.1.1.2. Brakeectomy

It is the total removal of the labial or lingual brake which aims to release the tension caused on the marginal gum or on the tongue. The procedure can be performed by conventional surgery, electrosurgery or laser.

2.1.2. Freinectomy: Conventional surgical technique [8,13].

Several techniques are used to perform the brakeectomy prior to the introduction of the laser technique in oral surgery.

Conventional brakeectomy was introduced by Archer (1961) and Kruger (1964).

It is a simple surgery, a diamond excision of the brake by a scalpel blade or a sharp instrument followed by stitches.

A periodontal dressing can be used to protect the wound. It should be changed weekly for 2 to 3 weeks.

This surgery can be heavy and can be time consuming especially for young patients. It depends on the skill of the practitioner on the one hand and the motivation of the patient on the other hand. Thus to have a complete healing, the patient must be motivated to have a rigorous hygiene. It is a very bloody act, which can be embarrassing and can compromise the good result and encourage recurrences. Some patients complain of post-operative discomfort. The appearance of pain and swelling in the days following the operation is not tolerated, especially in children in brake surgery.

2.1.3. Diode laser brakectomy [11,17]

The laser technique was developed very quickly.

The introduction of laser surgery, in recent years, shows a new alternative in the treatment that offers new perspectives due to these different characteristics.

It allows after a few seconds the realization of a precise and clean surgery.

It is a simple technique, with a short and reduced operating time and gives long-lasting results compared to conventional surgery.

2.1.4. The technique itself

The anaesthesia technique is no different from that used in the conventional technique, but the number of carpules required is reduced.

After an infiltration of the local anaesthetic, the diode laser is applied to the relevant brake. It allows a very fine cut, a bloodless release of the maxillary and/or mandibular brakes and to vaporize the entire fibrous tissue.

The laser moves parallel to the bone in order to avoid undesirable effects.

No surgical sutures are required, and no dressings are used after surgery, improving access for oral hygiene.

The risk of postoperative infection is reduced due to the sterilizing power of the laser.

The wound is left open. It will heal by a second intention healing by the production of granulation tissue and re-epithelization. This can be explained by the formation of the fibrin clot in the surgical wound which protects it from external irritation.

A favourable evolution is observed after 3 and 10 days.

Diode lasers have the advantage of a curative treatment without bleeding. It avoids untimely bleeding due to vascular rupture, which is comfortable for both patient and practitioner.

The best advantages of this procedure is that it shows no intraoperative complications with the absence of postoperative pain, oedema and swelling. Thus the prescription of analgesics is usually limited to the day of the operation and sometimes to the next half-day, which improves the patient's demand for these laser techniques in this type of operation.

2.2. Mouth ulcers and mouth ulcers

2.2.1. Canker sores

They are benign local ulcerations, of multifactorial origin, small in size, 1 to 9 mm in diameter, rounded or oval, well circumscribed, with clean edges with a yellowish background (fibrin), surrounded by an erythematous halo, evolving in 8 to 10 days.

Their appearance is preceded by prodromes: a localised redness with a tingling and burning sensation on which this ulceration will settle.

Although benign, they can be very painful, embarrassing and sometimes recurrent, leading the patient to seek emergency care.

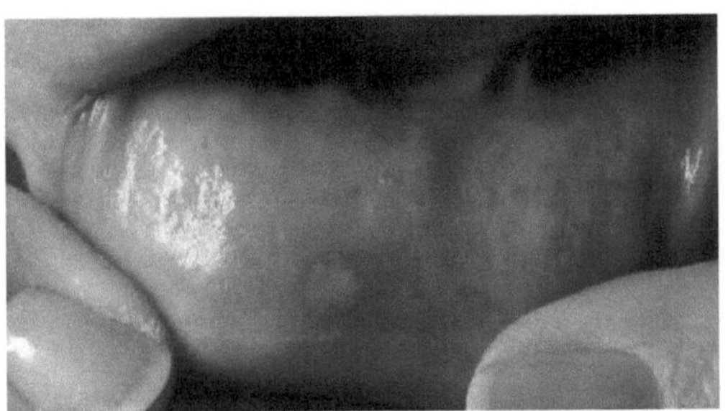

Figure 60: Aphthous ulceration. [9]

2.2.2. Conventional treatment of aphthous stomatitis [9,30]

Each form of aphthous stomatitis requires different treatment.

For mild forms of oral aphthosis, treatment is symptomatic. Symptoms can be reduced, but it is difficult to prevent recurrences. For minor forms, local treatment may be considered, such as topical application of local anaesthetics in gel or solution form to relieve pain before meals, acetylsalicylic acid 250 to 500mg, corticosteroids in local applications to attenuate the inflammatory component of these mouth ulcers, 0.2 or 0.1% mouthwashes or 1% gels based on an aqueous solution of chlorhexidine gluconate by continuous and prolonged use, to reduce the duration of the mouth ulcers and lengthen the periods of remission. For major forms, patients should be referred to specialists. Dietary measures are sometimes helpful.

Topical treatment	Systemic treatment	
Corticosteroids Sucralfate...	Specific	Non-specific
	VB12	Corticosteroids Colchicine Ciclosporin A...

2.2.3. Treatment of aphthous stomatitis by diode laser [30,42,44].

The diode laser is considered an alternative treatment method for the treatment of canker sores. It is more and more usable especially for recurrent forms.

A specific protocol must be followed.

After selecting the semiconductor laser parameters (power, frequency and wavelength), it is applied to the lesion for 3min divided into 4 sequences of 45s, with a rest phase of 15 to 20s between each session, at a distance of 2 to 3mm between the laser tip and the surface of the ulcer.

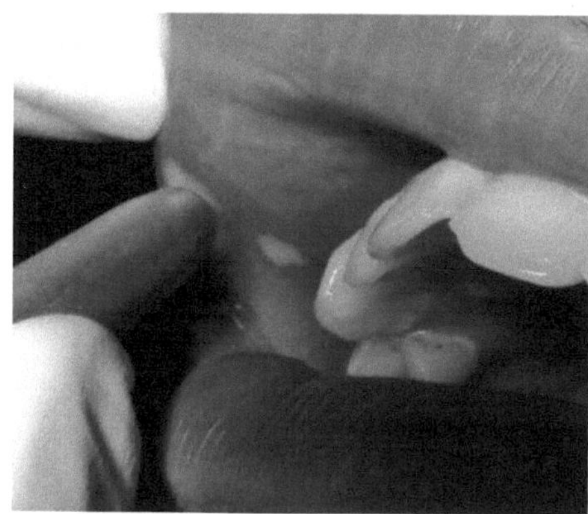

Figure 61: Treatment of aphthous stomatitis with diode laser. [29]

The patient thus shows immediate relief with the reduction of the extent of ulceration and the attenuation of all inflammatory phenomena.

After 3 days, rapid healing and complete resolution of aphthous stomatitis is achieved through increased blood flow and vasodilation of capillaries in the target tissues, which improves healing of these lesions and promotes tissue repair.

2.3 Oral herpes

2.3.1. Definition

These infections are common and most often mild.

The first lesions are characterized by the presence of small vesicles on an erythematous background in the oral mucosa, frequently accompanied by edema. After 2 to 3 days, these vesicles become pustules and a crust forms on the surface, sometimes causing pain. After a few days, the crust comes off, leaving scars.

Antiviral drugs such as acyclovir 5% cream may be beneficial if used at the onset of lesions. Because these agents have a relatively short half-life, they should be used several times during the day. The risk of drug nephrotoxicity should be considered for systemic administration. [19]

2.3.2. Diode laser treatment of herpes [14,19,47].

The laser treatment process is much simpler.

Its effect on the oral mucosa is twofold: an analgesic effect and a healing effect.

Its virucidal activity reduces or eliminates the need for routine prescribing of systemic antivirals.

In cases of initial infection and in the early stages of infection and even in the appearance of blisters and crusting in advanced stages, the laser is applied at a distance of 1 to 3 mm from the lesion.

Patients treated with the diode laser are all cured within the first 24 hours.

If the lesion is infected, the treatment lasts 3 to 4 days. No prescription medication is required.

Immediate considerable attenuation of the lesion during and after laser treatment with complete sedation of the symptomatology.

For recurrent forms, the diode laser is used to reduce the occurrence of recurrences. Thus, the annual period of recurrence appearance becomes much longer.

2.4. Gum surgery

2.4.1. The gingivectomy [3,22,37,40]

2.4.1.1. Definition

It is a surgical procedure that allows to reshape the gum and remove excess gum tissue, to have a better smile with an aesthetically harmonious gum contour that is compatible with individual and professional hygiene maneuvers.

Several surgical techniques are described such as internal and external bevel gingivectomy, electrosurgery...

These conventional surgeries can be followed by several complications such as intraoperative bleeding, postoperative pain, and scarring difficulties.

2.4.1.2. Diode laser gingivectomy

With the introduction of diode lasers, the surgical procedure becomes faster, painless and with optimal aesthetic results.

It allows the instantaneous removal of hyperplastic tissue and hypertrophic gingiva in a bloodless field with minimal or no postoperative pain.

No incision is necessary, the laser tip is held vertically at the marginal gum.

At the end of the surgery, about 1 mm of the depth of the gingival sulcus is preserved.

After reaching the ideal gingival contour with a good clinical crown height, the gum is cleaned with a cotton roll soaked in 3% hydrogen peroxide.

Compared to traditional surgical techniques, these advantages are numerous. It allows the practitioner to work in clean conditions with good haemostasis, it prevents damage to teeth and bones during the procedure due to its limited effects on soft tissues, it reduces the risk of postoperative infection, and it allows the patient to resume optimal hygiene within hours after surgery.

2.4.2. Gingival depigmentation [5,6,11,20]

2.4.2.1. Hyperpigmented gingiva: Definition

Gum colour can be an ethnic characteristic that differs from one individual to another and correlates with skin pigmentation. It is influenced by the vascularization of the gum, the thickness and degree of keratinization of the epithelium and the presence of pigmented cells (melanin) in the basal and supra-basal epithelial layer.

Several therapeutic modalities are used to treat it.

The most common technique is the surgical removal of unwanted pigmentation using scalpel blades. In this procedure, the gingival epithelium is surgically removed along with a layer of underlying connective tissue. The exposed connective tissue then heals in a second step.

2.4.2.2. Diode laser depigmentation

Currently, the treatment of gum hyperpigmentation using diode laser has gained popularity.

The protocol of use is very simple. Anaesthesia is not always necessary.

The diode laser was used in contact with the gum, acting on the melanocytes which are rich in melanin. In fact, it is easily absorbed by the soft tissues that contain melanins, hemoglobins and chromophores.

It is gently applied in a continuous mode.

Ablation begins with the mucco-gingival junction towards the free marginal gingiva and the interdental papilla.

After the [first] session, the stains will have a darker appearance. A white fibrin is formed after 24 hours, which will give way to a crust that will flake off after a few days.

In general, one to two laser sessions to treat hyperpigmentation is sufficient. Complete healing is completed after 10 days and the patient is extremely satisfied with normal gum colouring.

2.5. White lesions

2.5.1. White lesions of the oral cavity

These are common clinical lesions. They can represent a multitude of pathological processes ranging from a simple traumatic keratosis to a lesion with a potential for malignant transformation, or even squamous cell carcinoma.

Although often benign, some of these white lesions can become a site for the development of squamous cell carcinoma such as oral leukoplakia and lichen planus. [24]

2.5.2. Oral leukoplakia

2.5.2.1. Definition [35]

Oral leukoplakia is defined as "white plaque that cannot be characterized clinically or pathologically like any other disease" and is not associated with any other physical or chemical causative agent except smoking. It is the most common potentially malignant lesion of the oral mucosa. This may be due to the prolonged use of tobacco. It usually affects people over 40 years of age. It most often affects the lips, tongue, gums and oral floor. Overall prevalence varies from 0.5% to 3.4% and malignant transformation varies from 0.17% to 17.5%.

2.5.2.2. Conventional treatment of oral leukoplakia [31]

The therapeutic approach is related to the severity of the lesion, including its site, size and location with any associated dysplasia.

It is managed by a variety of treatment modalities, both medical and surgical.

Although there is no specific treatment to prevent its recurrence, giving up bad habits such as smoking and alcohol can reduce the likelihood of it recurring and turning into a malignant tumour.

Non-surgical, topical or systemic means (retinoids, vitamin A, bleomycin, ..) can be used. Various surgical treatment modalities have been recommended, including conventional surgery, cryotherapy, etc. These conventional surgeries are limited by the site and extent of the lesion.

2.5.2.3. Treatment of oral leukoplakia by diode laser [24,31,35].

By convention, the diode laser is considered an effective tool for the treatment of this pathology. It seems ideal, because of its innocuousness, ease of use and low morbidity:

- It is extremely effective in ablating leukoplakia.
- Post-operative complications associated with laser ablation are minimal.
- Pain is mild to moderate, with insignificant swelling for up to 72 hours after treatment.

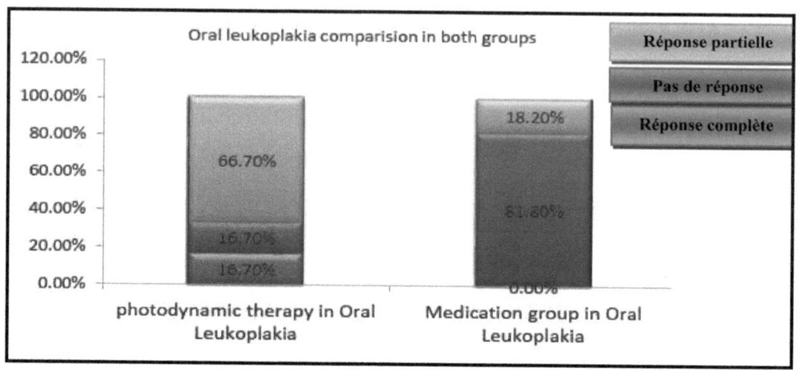

Figure 62: Comparison between conventional (drug) treatment and laser therapy. [24]

The advantages of laser therapy are its haemostatic potential and low tissue contraction, reduced postoperative pain, reduced swelling and peripheral inflammation, and reduced risk of infection.

2.5.3. The plan lichen

2.5.3.1. Definition [12]

Lichen planus is considered an autoimmune, chronic, mucocutaneous disease that can affect the skin, genital mucosa, nails, scalp and oral mucosa.

It is a keratotic lesion, of chronic evolution, manifests itself in several forms: reticular, papular, annular, linear, or plate-like. No definite etiology has been found, but it may be due to viral infections, stress or certain related drugs such as antihypertensives, oral hypoglycemic drugs, non-steroidal anti-inflammatory drugs, antiarrhythmics, etc.

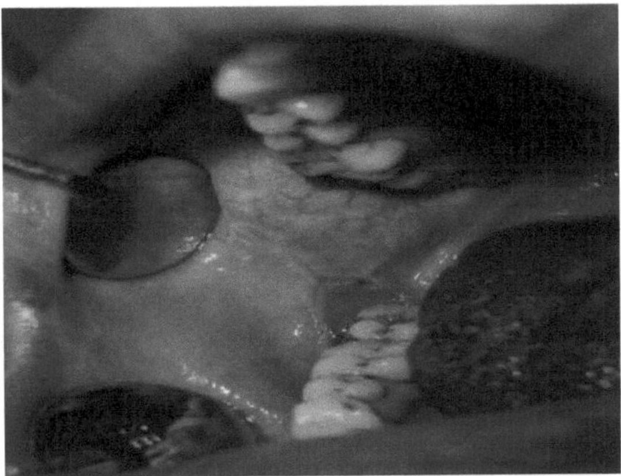

Figure 63: Mouth lichen at the level of the jugal mucosa. [28]

2.5.3.2. Conventional treatment of plane lichen [12].

Treatment of these chronic lesions is difficult.

We start by sanitizing the oral cavity by eliminating the local factors that promote it: poor oral hygiene, poorly fitting dentures and other traumatic factors...to reduce irritation.

But there is no cure for oral lichen planus.

Corticosteroids are sometimes prescribed. They are effective for erosive lesions that promote healing, but have no effect on reticular, papular or plaque lesions. Indeed, they help to reduce inflammatory signs, but may also promote the undesirable side effects of Candida Albican proliferation.

Because the lesions are diffuse, conventional surgery does not provide adequate results, therefore laser surgery is recommended as an alternative.

2.5.3.3. Diode laser treatment of plane lichen [28].

Conventional treatment of lichen planus based mainly on corticosteroids is a prolonged treatment and especially in case of recurrences, which in most cases cannot be avoided, and which depends on regular monitoring, which can lead to phenomena of dependency of patients on these drugs.

These corticosteroids prove their effectiveness in the treatment of erosive lesions, which is not the case for reticular forms and platelet lesions.

Similarly, they can reduce inflammation but for diffuse lesions they cannot give satisfactory results, until now, diode laser surgery is recommended as an advanced therapeutic alternative, which avoids the possible adverse effects caused by drugs.

It shows favourable clinical improvement of potentially malignant lesions with minimal side effects.

The procedure for its use is much simpler.

The site of the lesion is infiltrated with a local anesthetic. After protective measures have been taken, the lesion is removed by the application of a diode laser in direct contact with the injured mucosa.

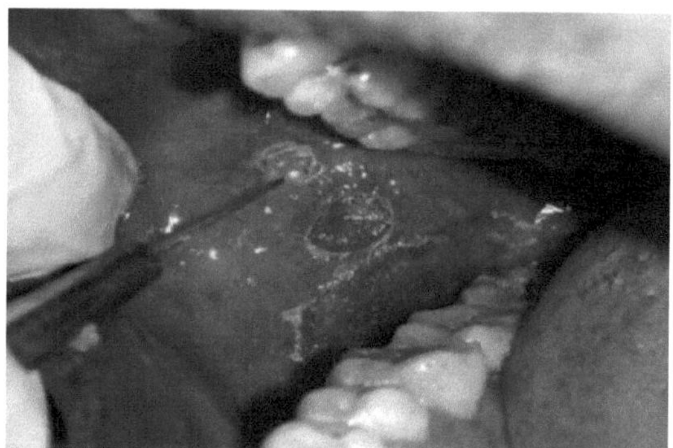

Figure 64: Irradiation of the damaged mucosa by diode laser. [35]

Damaged tissue is removed using a sterile gauge immersed in saline solution and this procedure is continued until the depth of the damaged tissue is reached. This laser causes a denaturation of the keratinocyte proteins of the superficial epithelium, resulting in the bleaching of the surgical site, which acts as a post-surgical dressing, reduces pain and improves healing with the least risk of secondary infection. A post-surgical anaesthetic gel may be prescribed for postoperative pain, as well as the application of ice packs to avoid oedema. A reduction in the extent of lesions and pain, as well as stable overall results, have generally been observed from the first session. Treatment is carried out twice a week for 2 months, and a complete remission of all symptoms is observed after 3 months.

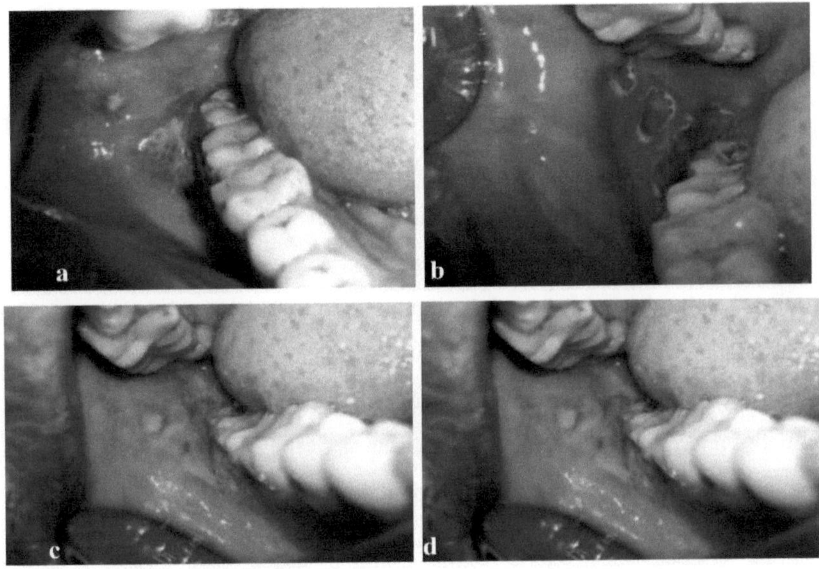

Figure 65: Flat lichen on the jugal mucosa: from right to left : (a) pre-operative photo, (b) immediate post-operative photo, (c) after one week, (d) after six weeks following diode laser irradiation. [35]

2.6. Benign tumours (Botryomycoma, fibroma, epulis...)

2.6.1. Definition

Benign tumours and pseudotumours of the oral mucosa represent an important variety of pathologies of the oral cavity that develop from epithelial cells and cells of the underlying connective tissue.

Their identification is based on their clinical aspects, the radiological examination as well as the histological aspect.

Gingival hypertrophy is a common clinical manifestation that evokes the diagnosis of a tumour lesion on clinical examination.

The pathogenesis and etiology of an enlarged gum depends on the radiological examination as well as the histological aspect of the lesion.

Several techniques are available to treat these oral lesions, including: surgical excision which is the most commonly used method, cryotherapy, electrosurgery and laser therapy... [18]

2.6.2. Treatment of benign tumors with diode laser [5,18,26].

After first confirming the clinical diagnosis of the nature of the lesion and its benign characteristic by biopsy, laser surgery is required.

Recently, the diode laser, in continuous or pulsed mode, has been used as a possible modality in oral surgery to excise benign tumours thanks to its photothermal and photoablative effect, while being at a distance from the oral mucosa and therefore no mechanical trauma to the surrounding tissues.

No medication is prescribed for the patient at the end of the surgery.

The major advantages of the application of the diode laser are relatively the control of bleeding, the reduction of the time of the surgical operation thus reducing the psychological trauma and panic of the patient, the immediate disinfection of the surgical wound, no sutures are necessary, no oedema and post-surgical pain, with optimal healing without after-effects.

2.7. Use of diode lasers in post-extarction [15,23,34].

Surgical removal of an impacted tooth (especially in the case of a lower wisdom tooth) is most often followed by postoperative pain and edema with jaw hypofunction.

Many factors contribute to these complex situations of discomfort, but the most important is the inflammatory process that is promoted by traumatic surgery.

After surgery, pain reaches its peak intensity 3 to 5 hours after surgery and persists for 2 to 3 days.

The edema reaches its maximum intensity in 12 to 48 hours, resolving between the fifth and seventh day.

These symptoms are generally alleviated by the prescription of analgesics, level two depending on the complexity of the procedure, corticosteroids and mouthwashes with antiseptic purpose.

Recently, the diode laser has been considered as an analgesic agent to control pain, and anti-inflammatory to limit inflammation and oedema as well as postoperative trismus with a real improvement in the postoperative period.

It also accelerates wound healing after extraction and bone regeneration.

It is applied intra-buccally at the extraction site 1 cm from the target tissue immediately after surgery for 2min.

2.8. Orthodontic traction of an impacted tooth

2.8.1. Definition

The prevalence of impacted teeth varies from 1% to 2.5% depending on the study population characteristics (gender, age, ethnicity).

Such a condition affects the maxillary arch more frequently, and the canines are the most affected teeth after the third molars. The inclusion of permanent teeth, especially in the front part of the dental arch, is both aesthetically and functionally disturbing.

Their repositioning on the arch is a multidisciplinary act that depends on good cooperation between surgery and orthodontics.

Surgical removal of the tooth is a critical step in the treatment plan to attach an orthodontic bracket.

The major disadvantage of this procedure is the bleeding during surgery which makes it difficult or impossible to glue the brackets to the vestibular surface of the tooth. [25,27]

2.8.2. Diode laser surgery [11,27]

Today, the diode laser is becoming an essential complement in many orthodontic procedures.

It easily removes soft tissue covering the crown of the impacted tooth and provides access for attachment and bonding of the orthodontic bracket without local anaesthesia.

The technique is simple. It starts with a biostimulation of the soft tissues covering the crown of the impacted tooth to reduce pain, using the laser in continuous emission, for 30 seconds.

The optical fibres are positioned vertically at a distance of 10mm from the target tissue.

Then, after brushing the alveolar mucosa facing the tooth with a cotton pad soaked in local anaesthetic for 30 seconds, an incision is created with the laser beam in pulsed emission according to sequences of 20 seconds separated by rest phases of 10 seconds. This procedure is completed after locating the crown of the impacted tooth. In this way, the surgical incision is widened in a centrifugal direction to create the necessary access to position and glue the orthodontic bracket in a clean and dry environment.

The enormous advantage of this technique is that it delimits a bloodless area to allow immediate and safe bonding of the orthodontic bracket.

The total duration of the surgical procedure was between 8 and 23 minutes.

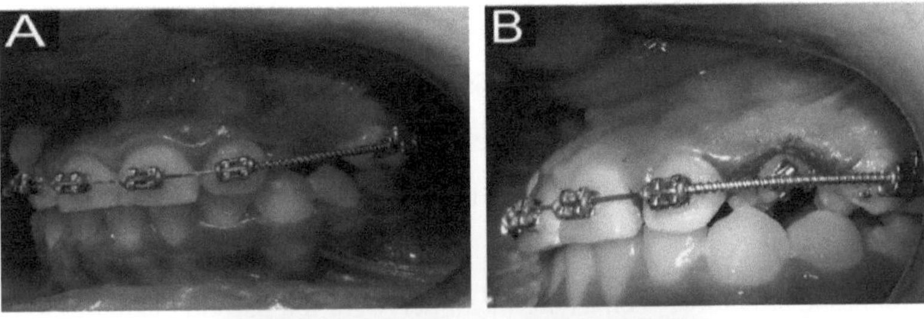
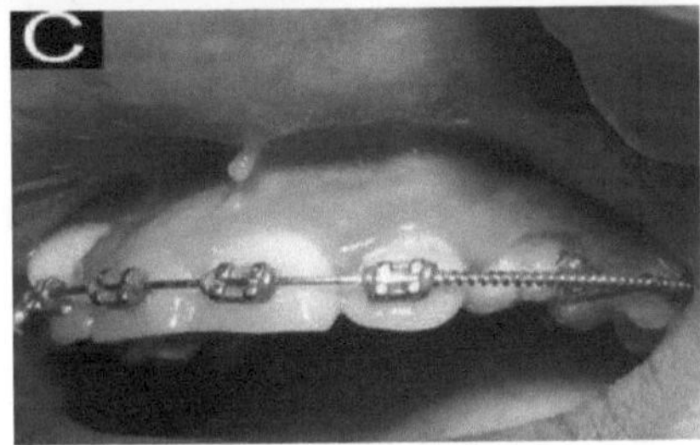

Figure 66: (A) maxillary canine included: (B) Immediately after 980 nm diode laser irradiation and immediate bonding of the gears, (C) postoperative photo after 10 days. [11]

2.9. Treatment of salivary gland pathology

2.9.1. Salivary lithiasis [21].

2.9.1.1. Definition

Salivary lithiasis is the most common benign condition of the salivary glands. It is characterized by the development of salivary stones that accumulate in the parenchyma of the salivary glands and associated excretory ducts, causing them to become obstructed.

In most cases, lithiasis is symptomatic, causing a painful swelling especially during a meal, also, these salivary stones can be a source of deep infection of the neck.

2.9.1.2. Conventional treatment

The goal of treatment for this benign condition is the restoration of normal salivary secretion. Its clinical management depends on the location and size of the salivary stones.

For small and medium size stones, the treatment is called conservative and aims to hydrate the salivary gland by taking sialagogues. But, generally, surgical removal of the stone is more tolerated by the patient.

For giant and intraglandular calculi, it is necessary in most cases to completely remove the gland transcutaneously, which is cumbersome, with risks for the surrounding structures such as the facial nerve for the parotid gland or the lingual nerve for the submandibular gland.

2.9.1.3. Treatment of salivary lithiasis by diode laser

Thanks to the diode laser, the treatment of salivary lithiasis becomes much simpler. It is a non-invasive therapeutic modality, minimally traumatic for the surrounding structures.

Irradiation of the excretory canal from the ostium to where the stone becomes visible, even allows the fragmentation of giant stones blocked either in the glandular parenchyma or in the excretory canal, without damaging the surrounding noble structures.

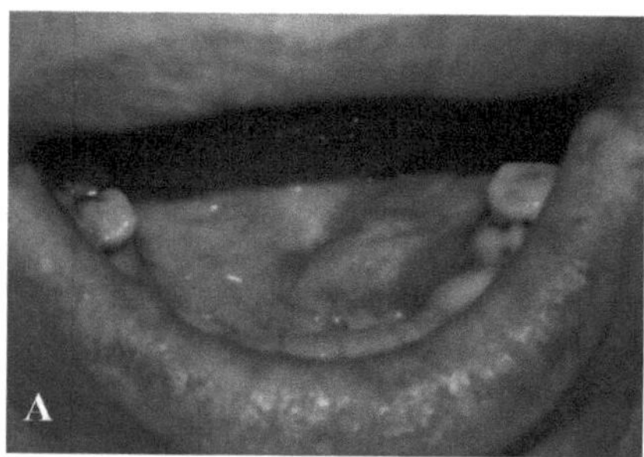

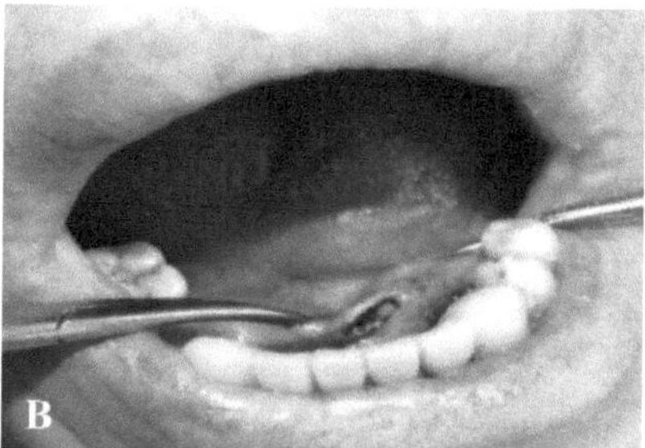

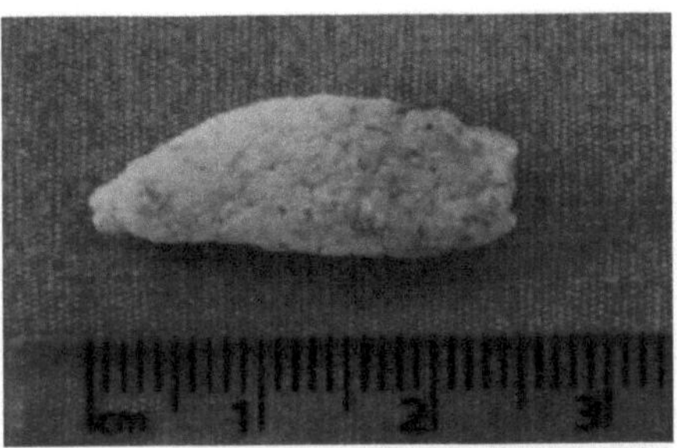

Figure 67: Salivary lithiasis in the sub-mandibular gland : (A) preoperative photo (endo-oral view), (B) incision of the mucous membrane around the lithiasis by diode laser, (C) giant salivary stone cleared from the warton canal. [21]

2.9.2. Mucoceles or mucoid cysts [1,33].

These are benign tumor pathologies of the accessory salivary glands of the oral mucosa. It is mainly due to mechanical trauma causing rupture of the ductal system of the accessory salivary glands and mucin spillage into the adjacent soft tissues.

These lesions are characterized by its bluish and transparent color, varying in size from 1-2mm to several centimeters.

The treatment of these mucoid cysts consists of surgical removal under local anaesthesia. Marsupialization may be indicated in retention cysts.

The diode laser is an easy to use technique. It allows by a precise photo-ablative action, thanks to the optical fibres, to make a circular incision all around the lesion.

It's less traumatic than conventional surgery, with less risk of recurrence.

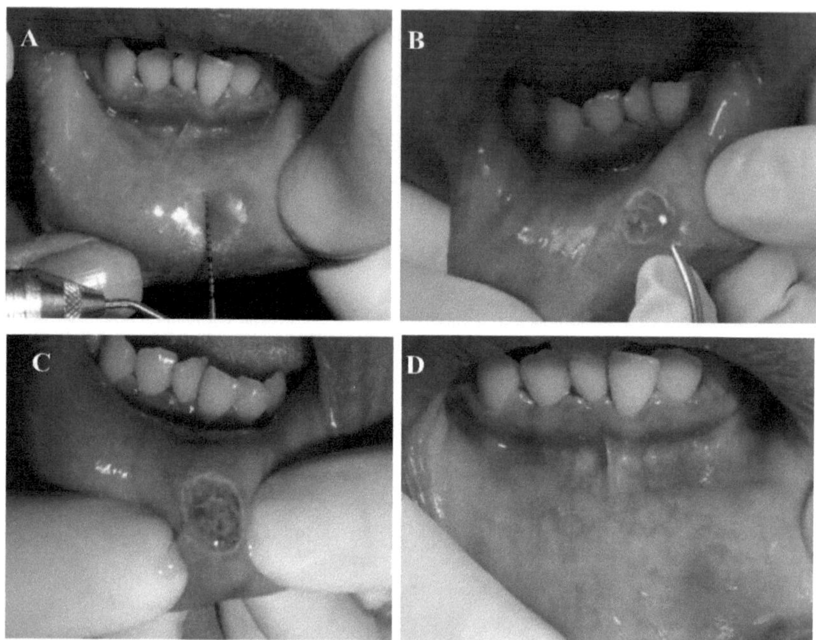

Figure 68: Mucocele in the lower labial mucosa: (A) preoperative photo, (B) excision of the lesion by diode laser in a contact mode, (C) immediate postoperative photo, (D) complete healing after 3 months. [1]

2.9.3. The frog [2,48]

It is a benign condition of the sublingual gland manifested by salivary retention at the oral floor level.

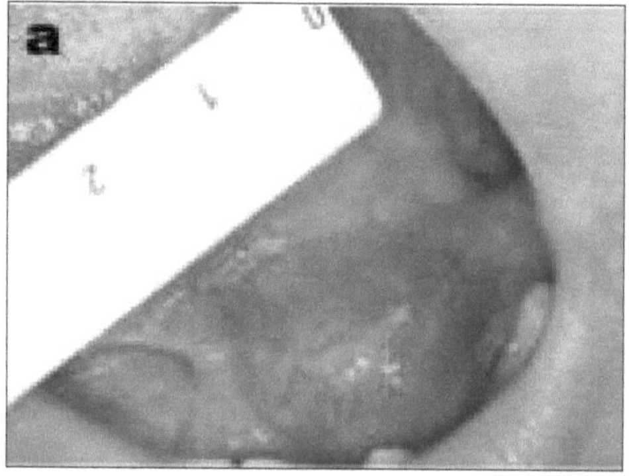

Figure 69: Salivary retention cyst at the oral floor: endo-oral view. [2]

The laser may be recommended because of the precision of the ablation, the sterile and clean surgical field and the low risk of damage to the Wharton canal and the nerves running through the gum.

2.10. Mucites induced by chemotherapy/radiotherapy [16,38,48].

2.10.1. Definition

Mucositis is a major and frequent complication induced by radiotherapy and/or chemotherapy in the treatment of cancers of the upper aerodigestive tract, characterized by the appearance of inflammatory erythematous areas associated with painful ulcerative patches and necrotic areas, even fractures in the advanced stages.

2.10.2. Conventional treatment of mucositis

No conservative or surgical treatment is effective in the long term.

Its management is most often symptomatic.

Depending on the patient's state of health, possible treatments include temporary or permanent discontinuation of bisphosphonates, prescription of mouthwashes with 1.4% sodium bicarbonate, use of systemic or local antibiotics or hyperbaric oxygen, and surgical debridement of lesions.

2.10.3 Diode laser treatment of mucositis

Laser phototherapy is a valuable aid in relieving this acute toxicity thanks to its analgesic and anti-inflammatory effects.

It is a promising, non-invasive technique, well tolerated by patients. It is administered for both preventive and curative purposes.

As a preventive measure, the diode laser stimulates the tissue repair process and prevents the development of severe mucositis, which improves the quality of life of patients undergoing chemotherapy by reducing the frequency of oral mucositis.

From a curative point of view, thanks to these photo-biological effects in the soft tissues, it triggers the activation of the local microcirculation of the irradiated areas, promoting increased fibroblastic activity and the development of capillaries, thus accelerating the healing process and improving healing even for grade 3 and 4 mucites.

2.11. Implantology: Peri-implantitis [7]

2.11.1. Definition

Peri-implantitis is an inflammatory *process of* the tissues around an osseointegrated implant with the loss of bone support, which limits the longevity of the implant-supported prosthesis.

2.11.2. Conventional treatment of peri-implantitis

Peri-implantitis is treated by mechanical techniques by debridement of the bone defect and decontamination of the implant surface with carbon fiber curettes, and chemical techniques by prescribing antimicrobial agents to control microorganisms in most of the pockets around the implants.

In clinical practice, difficulties are sometimes encountered in cleaning between the implant coils, which are always narrower than the tip of the ultrasound insert or titanium curette.

Similarly, the use of antimicrobial agents and the need to use different antibiotics due to the diversity of periodontopathogenic bacteria can lead to an increase in the number of bacteria resistant to these agents and sometimes create adverse reactions.

Considering all these complications, the diode laser is involved as an alternative technique.

2.11.3 Treatment of peri-implantitis by diode laser

It is a new non-invasive technique, which meets the mechanical requirements of decontamination of the implant microsurface and seems to give good results. It has a bactericidal effect on the peri-implant flora, by eliminating infiltrated bacteria and potentiating healing, without damaging the implant surface.

The operating protocol is simple and fast. The laser beam is directed to the pockets in 3 steps as follows:

1. Transgingival irradiation.
2. Direct irradiation in the pocket with a circular movement.
3. Removal of granulation tissue from the infected pouch in areas difficult to treat by conventional means with a circular motion.

3. Diode laser limits [10,11,41,51].

Although the diode laser is much cheaper than other types of lasers, it is still more expensive than conventional surgical techniques.

This high cost is related to the training courses programmed for these various clinical applications to allow optimal use and improve the positive effects of the diode laser.

Indeed, before any clinical application, a basic knowledge of physics, physiology, wavelengths, their interactions with tissue and their applications, as well as evidence-based experience is required.

Thus, training on the clinical applications of lasers is necessary to be successful in choosing the appropriate parameters during diode laser surgery.

The diode laser can be used to treat almost all small to medium soft tissue lesions. For larger lesions, other laser systems or conventional methods are recommended.

4. Precautions when using the diode laser and protective measures [51].

The laser beam can damage the retina and the lens of the eye. A direct beam will cause permanent damage. Reflected beams can also cause damage to the practitioner, patient and assistants.

Most laser beams are invisible to the human eye, which makes them dangerous. Each person who views the laser beam directly must wear protective eyewear specially designed for particular wavelengths and the device being used.

Conclusion

A oday, diode lasers have an undeniable place in oral medicine and surgery.

It acts deep in the soft tissues thanks to these wavelengths, which are highly penetrating in tissues rich in haemoglobin and melanin, without any risk to the hard tissues.

This innovative, non-invasive method is well exploited in soft tissue surgeries such as brakeectomy, gum depigmentation, treatment of white lesions and benign tumors .

It allows the practitioner to ablate different soft tissue lesions and perform the necessary tissue corrections with less post-operative follow-up thanks to its analgesic and anti-inflammatory effect, with improved healing without any sequelae or recurrences, in optimal conditions of comfort compared to conventional surgical techniques.

However, in order to achieve repeatable results and enhance positive effects, a basic knowledge of physics, physiology, wavelengths, their interactions with tissue and their applications, as well as evidence-based experience is required prior to any clinical application.

And finally, thanks to these well-controlled parameters, which can be adjusted according to the clinical situation and the target tissues involved, the diode laser allows a wide range of indications not only in oral surgery, but also in other disciplines of dentistry such as periodontology, pedodontics, implantology, endodontics and dental prosthesis.

References

1. **Ahad A, Tandon S, Lamba AK, Faraz F, Anand P, Aleem A.**
   Diode laser assisted excision and low level laser therapy in the
   management of mucus extravasation cysts: a case series.
   J Lasers Med Sci 2017;8(3):155-9.

2. **Amaral MB, Freitas IZ, Pretel H, Abreu MH, Mesquita RA.**
   Low level laser effect after micro-marsupialization technique in treating
   ranulas and mucoceles: a case series report.
   Lasers Med Sci 2012;27(6):1251-5.

3. **Asnaashari M, Azari-Marhabi S, Alirezaei S, Asnaashari N.**
   Clinical application of 810nm diode laser to remove gingival hyperplasic
   lesion.
   J Lasers Med Sci 2013;4(2):96-8.

4. **Asnaashari M, Safavi N.**
   Application of low level lasers in dentistry (Endodontic).
   J Lasers Med Sci 2013;4(2):57-66.

5. **Azma E, Safavi N.**
   Diode laser application in soft tissue oral surgery.
   J Lasers Med Sci 2013;4(4):206-11.

6. **Bakutra G, Shankarapillai R, Mathur L, Manohar B.**
   Comparative evaluation of diode laser ablation and surgical stripping
   technique for gingival depigmentation: A clinical and
   immunohistochemical study.
   Int J Health Sci 2017;11(2):51-8.

7. **Birang E, Talebi Ardekani MR, Rajabzadeh M, Sarmadi G, Birang R, Gutknecht N.**

Evaluation of effectiveness of photodynamic therapy with low-level diode laser in nonsurgical treatment of peri-implantitis.

J Lasers Med Sci 2017;8(3):136-42.

8. **Brookes A, Bowley DM.**

Tongue tie: The evidence for frenotomy.

Early Hum Dev 2014;90:765-8.

9. **Cui RZ, Bruce AJ, Rogers RS.**

Recurrent aphthous stomatitis.

Clin Dermatol 2016;34(4):475-81.

10. **David CM, Gupta P.**

Lasers in dentistry: a review.

Int J Adv Health Sci 2010;2(8) :7-13.

11. **Derikvand N, Chinipardaz Z, Ghasemi S, Chiniforush N.**

The versatility of 980 nm diode laser in dentistry: a case series.

J Lasers Med Sci 2016;7(3):205-8.

12. **Derikvand N, Ghasemi SS, Moharami M, Shafiei E, Chiniforush N.**

Management of oral lichen planus by 980 nm diode laser.

J Lasers Med Sci 2017;8(3):150-4.

13. **Devishree G, Gujjari SK, Shubhashini PV.**

Frenectomy: A Review with the reports of surgical techniques.

J Clin Diagn Res 2012;6(9):1587-92.

14. **Donnarumma G, De Gregorio V, Fusco A et al.**

Inhibition of HSV-1 replication by laser diode irradiation: possible mechanism of action.

Int J Immunopathol Pharmacol 2010;23(4):1167-76.

15. **Ferrante M, Petrini M, Trentini P, Perfetti G, Spoto G.**

Effect of low-level laser therapy after extraction of impacted lower third molars.

Lasers Med Sci 2013;28(3):845-9.

16. **Freire Mdo R, Freitas R, Colombo F, Valença A, Marques AM, Sarmento VA.**

LED and laser photobiomodulation in the prevention and treatment of oral mucositis: experimental study in hamsters.

Clin Oral Investig 2014;18(3):1005-13.

17. **Gargari M, Autili N, Petrone A, Prete V.**

Using the diode laser in the lower labial frenum removal.

Oral Implantol 2012;5(2-3):54-7.

18. **Ghadimi S, Chiniforush N, Najafi M, Amiri S.**

Excision of epulis granulomatosa with diode laser in 8 years old boy.

J Lasers Med Sci 2015;6(2):92-5.

19. **Honarmand M, Farhadmollashahi L, Vosoughirahbar E.**

Comparing the effect of diode laser against acyclovir cream for the treatment of herpes labialis.

J Clin Exp Dent 2017 ;9(6):729-32.

20. **Jha N, Ryu JJ, Wahab R, Al-Khedhairy AA, Choi EH, Kaushik NK.**

Treatment of oral hyperpigmentation and gummy smile using lasers and role of plasma as a novel treatment technique in dentistry: An introductory review.

Oncotarget 2017;8(12):20496-509.

21. **Kilinc Y, Cetiner S.**

Surgical removal of a giant sialolith by diode laser.

Open J Stomatol 2014;4:484-8.

22. **Kumar P, Rattan V, Rai S.**

Comparative evaluation of healing after gingivectomy with electrocautery and   laser.

J Oral Biol Craniofac Res 2015;5(2):69-74.

23. **López-Ramírez M, Vílchez-Pérez MA, Gargallo-Albiol J, Arnabat-Domínguez J, Gay-Escoda C.**

Efficacy of low-level laser therapy in the management of pain, facial swelling, and postoperative trismus after a lower third molar extraction. A preliminary study.

Lasers Med Sci 2012;27(3):559-66.

24. **Maloth KN, Velpula N, Kodangal S et al.**

Photodynamic therapy – a non-invasive treatment modality for precancerous lesions.

J Lasers Med Sci 2016;7(1):30-6.

25. **Manne P, Zakkula S, Atla J, Muvva SB, Sampath A.**

Redefining smile-a multidisciplinary approach.

J Clin Diagn Res 2013;7(7):1527-9.

26. **Mathur E, Sareen M, Dhaka P, Baghla P.**

Diode laser excision of oral benign lesions.

J Lasers Med Sci 2015;6(3):129-32.

27. **Migliario M, Rizzi M, Lucchina AG, Renò F.**

Diode laser clinical efficacy and mini-invasivity in surgical exposure of impacted teeth.

J Craniofac Surg 2016;27(8):779-84.

28. **Misra N, Chittoria N, Umapathy D, Misra P.**

Efficacy of diode laser in the management of oral lichen planus.

BMJ Case Rep 2013;1:1-15.

29. **Misra N, Maiti D, Misra P, Singh AK.**

940 nm diode laser therapy in management of recurrent apthous ulcer.

BMJ Case Rep 2013;2013. pii: bcr2012008489.

30. **Nasry SA, El Shenawy HM, Mostafa D, Ammar NM.**

Different modalities for treatment of recurrent aphthous stomatitis. A Randomized clinical trial.

J Clin Exp Dent 2016 ;8(5):517-22.

31. **Natekar M, Raghuveer HP, Rayapati DK et al.**

A comparative evaluation: Oral leukoplakia surgical management using diode laser, CO2 laser, and cryosurgery.

J Clin Exp Dent 2017;9(6):779-84.

32. **Para A.**

Illustration of diode and Nd-YAG laser effects in endodontics and surgery.

Actual Odontostomatol 2015;272:15-22.

33. **Ramkumar S, Ramkumar L, Malathi N, Suganya R.**

Excision of mucocele using diode laser in lower lip.

Case Rep Dent 2016;2016:1-4.

34. **Rani A, Mohanty S, Sharma P, Dabas J.**

Comparative evaluation of ER:CR:YSGG, diode laser and alvogyl in the management of alveolar osteitis: a prospective randomized clinical study.

J Maxillofac Oral Surg 2016;15(3):349-54.

35. **Reddy Kundoor VK, Patimeedi A, Roohi S, Maloth KN, Kesidi S, Masabattula GK.**

Efficacy of diode laser for the management of potentially malignant disorders.

J Lasers Med Sci 2015;6(3):120-3.

36. **Rey G, Missika P.**

Lasers and dental surgery binnovations and clinical strategies.

Paris: CdP, 2010.

37. **Shankar BS, Reddy PS, Saritha G, Reddy JM.**

Chronic inflammatory gingival overgrowths: laser gingivectomy &
gingivoplasty.

J Int Oral Health 2013;5(1):83-7.

38. **Silva GB, Sacono NT, Othon-Leite AF et al.**

Effect of low-level laser therapy on inflammatorymediator release during
chemotherapy-induced oral mucositis: a randomized preliminary study.

Lasers Med Sci 2015;30(1):117-26.

39. **Singh SC, Zeng HB, Guo C, Cai W.**

Lasers: fundamentals, types, and operations. In : Singh ,H.B.
Zeng,Chunlei Guo,Weiping Cai, eds. Nanomaterials: processing and
characterization with lasers.

Weinheim : Wiley-VCH, 2012:34-41.

40. **Sobouti F, Rakhshan V, Chiniforush N, Khatami M.**

Effects of laser-assisted cosmetic smile lift gingivectomy on postoperative
bleeding and pain in fixed orthodontic patients: a controlled clinical trial.

Prog Orthod 2014;15:66.

41. **Stubinger S, Saldamli B, Jurgens P, Ghazal G, Zeilhofer H.**

Soft tissue surgery with diode laser - theoretical and clinical aspects.

Rev Mens Switzerland Odontostomatol 2006;116(8):818.

42. **Suter VG, Sjölund S, Bornstein MM.**

Effect of laser on pain relief and wound healing of recurrent aphthous
stomatitis: a systematic review.

Lasers Med Sci 2017;32(4):953-63.

43. **Tachmatzidis T, Dabarakis N.**

Only lasers can be used for low level laser therapy.

Balk J Dent Med 2016; 20:131-7.

44. **Vale FA, Moreira MS, de Almeida FC, Ramalho KM.**
Low-level laser therapy in the treatment of recurrent aphthous ulcers: a systematic review.
Sci World J 2015;2015:1-7.

45. **Verma SK, Maheshwari S, Singh RK, Chaudhari PK.**
Laser in dentistry: An innovative tool in modern dental practice.
Natl J Maxillofac Surg 2012; 3(2):124-32.

46. **Vizo K, Malhotra P, Sonia PO, Arora N.**
Diode laser: "bloodless" boon for soft tissue surgery in periodontics.
J Appl Dent Med Sci 2016;2(4):57-62.

Internet references:

47. **Alfonso G, Muzoz PJ.**
Laser therapy of human herpes: Simplex lesions [Online].
Retrieved March 19, 2018], available from the URL:
http://www.sld.cu/galerias/pdf/sitios/rehabilitacion-
fis/laser_y_herpers_simple.pdf

48. **Batista-Cruzado A, Torres-Lagares D, Moreno-Manteca B et al.**
Laser in Oral Medicine and Surgery Part II [Online].
[Accessed on 29/04/2018], available from URL: https://www.dental-
tribune.com/epaper/ce-magazines/laser-france-archived/laser-france-no-
1-2013-0113-[18-22].pdf

49. **Gaultier F.**
Contribution of lasers in oral surgery [Online].
Accessed on 08/04/2018], available from URL:
https://www.researchgate.net/publication/283257232_Apport_des_lasers
_en_chirurgie_buccale

50. **Goldstep F.**

   Diode lasers: the soft tissue handpiece [Online].

   Accessed on 24/04/2018], available from URL: https://www.dental-tribune.com/epaper/ce-magazines/laser-france-archived/laser-france-no-2-2012-0212-[38-40].pdf

51. **Graeber JJ.**

   Diode Lasers: A Primer [Online].

   [Accessed 12/02/2018], available from URL: https://www.dentalacademyofce.com/courses/2564/PDF/1401ceiGraeber_rev3.pdf.

52. **Schwob C, Julien L.**

   The laser: principle of operation [Online].

   [Accessed 12/04/2018], available from URL: https://www.refletsdelaphysique.fr/articles/refdp/pdf/2010/04/refdp20102 1p12.pdf

Contents

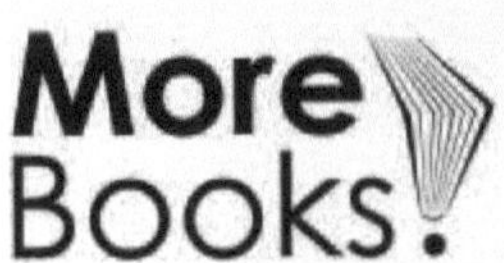

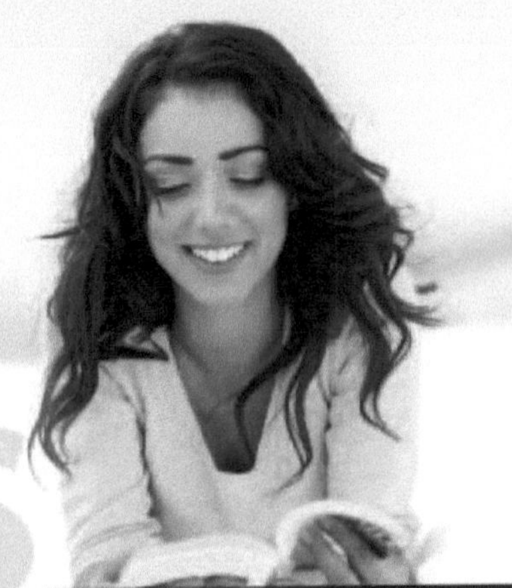

yes
I want morebooks!

Buy your books fast and straightforward online - at one of world's fastest growing online book stores! Environmentally sound due to Print-on-Demand technologies.

Buy your books online at
www.morebooks.shop

Kaufen Sie Ihre Bücher schnell und unkompliziert online – auf einer der am schnellsten wachsenden Buchhandelsplattformen weltweit! Dank Print-On-Demand umwelt- und ressourcenschonend produziert.

Bücher schneller online kaufen
www.morebooks.shop

KS OmniScriptum Publishing
Brivibas gatve 197
LV-1039 Riga, Latvia
Telefax: +371 686 204 55

info@omniscriptum.com
www.omniscriptum.com

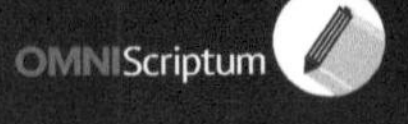